THE INDIAN OPERATION OF

COUCHING

FOR CATARACT

THE INDIAN OPERATION OF COUCHING FOR CATARACT

INCORPORATING

THE HUNTERIAN LECTURES

ROBERT HENRY ELLIOT

GYAN

Published by

GYAN

Gyan Publishing House
5, Ansari Road
Daryaganj, New Delhi-110002
Phone: 011-47034999, 9811692060
E-mail: books@gyanbooks.com

Distribution Network
gyanbooks.com
India, USA, Canada, UK, Australia, France

ISBN:978-81-212-9136-1 (PB)
First Published, 1918

2nd Impression 2023

Printed at: Gyan Press, Delhi.

THE INDIAN OPERATION OF COUCHING FOR CATARACT
AUTHOR: ROBERT HENRY ELLIOT

PLATE I.

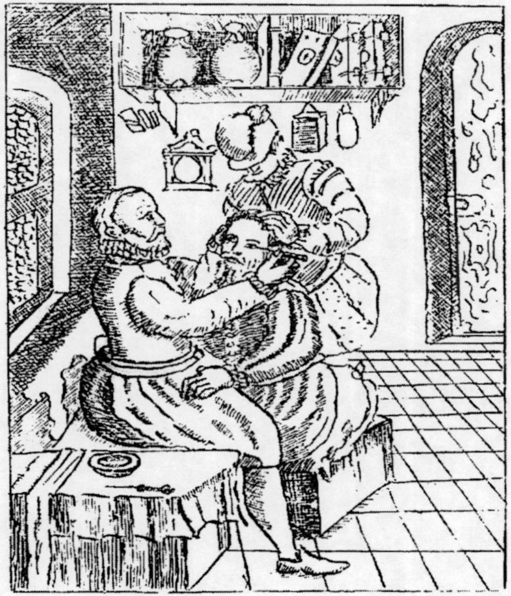

Copied by C. A. R. H.

FIG. 1.—The positions of the patient, operator, and assistant, as depicted by Bartisch (Albertotti).

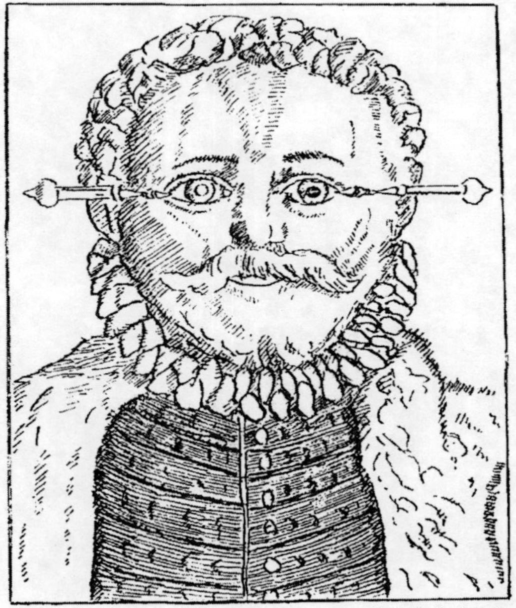

Copied by C. A. R. H.

FIG. 2.—To illustrate the method of introducing the needle in Bartisch's operation (Albertotti). The cataract is *in situ* in the right eye, and couched in the left eye.

THE INDIAN OPERATION OF COUCHING FOR CATARACT

INCORPORATING

THE HUNTERIAN LECTURES

DELIVERED BEFORE THE ROYAL COLLEGE OF SURGEONS OF ENGLAND ON FEBRUARY 19 AND 21, 1917

BY

ROBERT HENRY ELLIOT

M.D., B.S. LOND., SC.D. EDIN., F.R.C.S. ENG., ETC.
LIEUT.-COLONEL I.M.S. (RETIRED)
LATE SUPERINTENDENT OF THE GOVERNMENT OPHTHALMIC HOSPITAL, MADRAS;
LATE PROFESSOR OF OPHTHALMOLOGY, MEDICAL COLLEGE, MADRAS; AND LATE FELLOW OF THE UNIVERSITY OF MADRAS;
HONORARY FELLOW OF THE AMERICAN ACADEMY OF OPHTHALMOLOGY AND OTOLARYNGOLOGY.

WITH 45 ILLUSTRATIONS

PAUL B. HOEBER
67 & 69 EAST 59TH STREET
NEW YORK
1918

To

E. TREACHER COLLINS, Esq., F.R.C.S. ENG.,

IN GRATEFUL ACKNOWLEDGMENT OF THE ASSISTANCE WHICH HIS WORK ON THE PATHOLOGY OF THE EYE HAS BEEN TO ALL WHO DESIRE TO ADVANCE THE SCIENCE OF OPHTHALMOLOGY

PREFACE

It is a quarter of a century since I first landed in India. In common with very many other surgeons, my attention was early attracted to the operation of couching as performed by its Indian exponents, and I was horrified to see how bad the majority of the results were. It appeared to me that the outstanding need was for carefully compiled statistics, in order that a fair judgment might be formed on the subject. I divested my mind of partisanship and bias, and sought every opportunity to discuss the method and its results with anyone and everyone whose knowledge was likely to be of use to me in my quest, whether they were laymen or surgeons, Europeans or Indians, officials or non-officials. The office of Superintendent of the Government Ophthalmic Hospital, Madras, afforded an unrivalled field for work, and the staff of the hospital co-operated with me in a manner which I find it impossible to acknowledge suitably. My thanks are especially due to Lieutenant H. C. Craggs, Assistant-Surgeon C. Taylor, and Dr. Ekambaram, for the valuable help they gave me. After I left India, Captain W. C. Gray acted for me as Superintendent, and later Major H. Kirkpatrick succeeded me permanently. Both of these officers most generously placed the material of the hospital still at my disposal, and rendered me very valuable service in the study of my subject. The great majority of the microscopic slides were very beautifully prepared for me by Mr. W. Chesterman. I am also indebted to Mr. S. Stephenson and Mr. A. C. Hudson for very kindly sectioning some of the globes for me. The photographs, both macroscopic and microscopic, were taken by Mrs. Elliot, without whose help I could not have written the book. Mr. E. Treacher Collins has generously given me advice and assistance of the greatest value in the study of a number of the preparations, and I have acted freely on the suggestions he has been good enough to make. I desire to express to the Council of the Royal College of Surgeons of England my acknowledgment of the honour they conferred on me by electing me to a Hunterian Professorship of the College. By the kindness of the authorities concerned, I have been enabled to include in this book articles which have appeared in the *Lancet*, in the *Ophthalmic Record*, and in the Proceedings of the Ophthalmological Society of the United Kingdom.

The collection of fifty-four eyeballs, on which the work for my Hunterian Lectures was founded, I have had the honour to present to the Museum of the Royal College of Surgeons. I think I am justified in claiming that it is unrivalled, and likely to remain so. At the suggestion of Sir John Bland-Sutton, I have endeavoured so to write the chapter on pathology that it may furnish a guide to any who care to study the subject within the walls of that museum. At the same time, I have striven to make it readable and of interest to those who have no such opportunity. In this the photographs have greatly helped me.

As I have already said, I have given nearly a quarter of a century's intermittent work to elucidate these problems, which I felt were of wide interest, not merely to India or to the East alone, but to the whole civilized world. During the last two years I have devoted a very large proportion of my spare time continuously to the subject, but it is so immense and so far-reaching that I feel I have left much unfinished. On every hand fresh problems open up, till there seems no limit to what might be done, given time and opportunity. This operation of couching, so old that its origin is lost in the dim mists of antiquity, has still much that is new to be learnt for the seeking. There are many of the younger surgeons in the East who could carry the work much farther if they would, and who would be a hundred-fold repaid if they did. Will they?

ROBERT HENRY ELLIOT.

54, WELBECK STREET,
CAVENDISH SQUARE, W.,
1917.

CONTENTS

LIST OF ILLUSTRATIONS

PLATE IV.

PLATE V.

PLATE VI.

PLATE VII.

COUCHING FOR CATARACT

CHAPTER I

THE HISTORY OF COUCHING

THE operation of couching for cataract is one of the most ancient procedures known to surgery, the earliest description of the method being that given by Celsus, a contemporary of Christ's. The first historical mention of ophthalmic surgeons was in Alexandria, at the time when medicine and surgery underwent separation from each other in that great and flourishing city, nearly three centuries before the dawn of the Christian era, and Galen states that some of these surgeons devoted themselves exclusively to operating on cataracts. Celsus speaks of the writings of a famous Alexandrian surgeon, named Philoxenes, who lived 270 years before Christ, and from whom he apparently derived much of his lore. These writings have unfortunately been lost, thus yielding to Celsus the proud position of being the first author whose description of the operation has come down to modern times. Sprengel is of the opinion that couching was not only known long before the time of Celsus, but also that the technique of the operation, even at that distant era, varied widely in the hands of its different exponents. Of the correctness of this view there can be little doubt. Sir John Bland-Sutton has recently published a most interesting memoir on the recovery of the sight of Tobit at the hands of his son Tobias, as described in the Apocrypha, and has included in it a copy of Rembrandt's picture of the famous operation. Whether the displacement of the lens was due to the rubbing employed or to more definite operative measures must be left to speculation, but, in considering this point, it is worth remembering that the Eastern coucher of to-day hides the fact that he is performing an operation under the cloak of the application of a medicinal paste. Nor must we forget that the anointing of the eyes of the blind with clay played a leading part in one at least of the New Testament miracles, and is suggested in a second. It is to be remembered that the Founder of Christianity took His examples from, and moulded His teachings by the aid of things familiar to the people in their everyday life. The influence of the Oriental on the introduction of couching to the Western surgeon is shown by the repeated references in the history of the subject to Eastern exponents of the procedure. Thus, Razes speaks of the work of an Indian named Tabri, and Avicenna, himself an Arabian, describes at length the instruments and technique of the Arab cataract operators. Abu El Kasim's name proclaims his Arab parentage, despite the fact that he is spoken of as a Spanish surgeon, and the conviction is deepened by the fact that he spoke of the Arabs in Spain as confining themselves to couching in the treatment of cataract, showing he was in intimate touch with them. Nor must we forget to mention the work of Haly Abbas, and of his distinguished son Jesu Haly.

When we endeavour to ascertain the probable date of the first invention of the operation in the East, the fog of uncertainty closes down over us, obliterates all trace of our quest, and drives us to fall back on inference. Those who have spent their lives in an Eastern land know the unbending force of tradition, the hereditary character of occupations, and the intense conservatism of Oriental peoples. All these influences are against change of any kind, and greatly retard the spread of new ideas. When we consider an operation like couching, which is well known over the whole of the East, and which meets in the simplest manner an age-long need, felt in every village of a tropical or subtropical country, it is not difficult to believe that the procedure may have been one of the early fruits of advancing civilisation, far away back in Babylon the Great, or even earlier still in the home of the Pyramids, tens of centuries before the dawn of the Christian era. From these attractive speculations we must return to weigh the literature of our subject, of which the foundation was so well and truly laid by the great Celsus. His description of the technique he employed is as follows:

"Before the operation the patient must use a spare diet. . . . After this preparation he must sit in a light place, in a seat facing the light, and the physician must sit opposite the patient on a seat a little higher; an assistant behind taking hold of the patient's head, and keeping it immovable, for the sight may be lost for ever by a slight motion. Moreover, the eye itself must be rendered more fixed by laying wool upon the other and tying it on. The operation must be performed on the left eye by the right hand, and on the right by the left hand. Then the needle, sharp-pointed, but by no means too slender, is to be applied and must be thrust in, but in a straight direction, through the two coats, in the middle part betwixt the black of the eye and the external angle opposite to the middle of the cataract. . . . The needle must be turned upon the cataract and gently moved up and down there, and by degrees work the cataract downward below the pupil; when it has passed the pupil, it must be pressed down with a considerable force that it may settle in the inferior part."

Further details follow. To put the matter shortly in modern terminology, Celsus introduced a needle through the sclera and choroid into the vitreous chamber, and depressed the lens from behind, after first rupturing its posterior capsule by vertical strokes made with the point of the instrument. As already mentioned, Galen (born A.D. 131) states that there were both in Alexandria and in Rome surgeons who confined themselves to operating upon cataract. Apparently he also described his own procedure, for some five centuries later Paulus Ægineta (*circa* A.D. 630), in detailing his technique, gave Galen the credit for it. There is practically no difference between the method they both employed and that originally laid down by Celsus. A point of real interest in this connection is that the description of the operation given by Paulus is practically the only one extant from the pen of a Greek author, though not a few of them mention couching and advocate it.

For the next landmark in the study of the subject we have to pass over three and a half centuries, till we come to the writings of Avicenna (*circa* A.D. 980), in which we find introduced a new feature in the technique; for he mentions that the Arab surgeons used two instruments for couching—viz., a two-edged lancet with which they made a corneal incision, and a needle with which they depressed the cataract, after introducing it through the incision thus made. In this needle there was an eye near the point, through which a thread was inserted. According to Avicenna, the object of this was to help depress the lens, but it seems at least possible that the thread passed through this eye was wound round the instrument, and so served as a stop, similar to that used by the Indian coucher to-day. In any case the description is of great interest, linking as it does the Mahomedan operator of the twentieth century with his predecessor of the tenth. The famous Spanish surgeon Abu El Kasim adopted exactly the same technique for couching as that we have just described. This, as has already been suggested, is not in the least remarkable, for his name bespeaks his Arab descent.

The next description of the operation, which claims our interest, is that by Benvenuto (Benevenutus Hyerosolimitamus), who flourished in the twelfth century. The quaint blending of religion and science, which it reveals, makes it very attractive reading: "Towards the third hour, the patient having fasted, thou shouldst make him sit astride of an ordinary chair, and thou shouldst sit before him in the same way. Keep the good eye of the patient shut, and begin to operate on the bad eye, in the name of Jesus Christ. With one hand raise the upper lid, and with the other hold the silver needle, and place it in the part where the small angle of the eye is. Perforate the same covering of the eye, turning the instrument round and round between the fingers, till thou hast touched with the point of the needle that putrid water which the Arabs and Saracens called Mesoret, and which we call cataract. Then beginning from the upper part, remove it from the place where it is before the pupil, and make it come down in front, and then hold it for as long as it takes to say four or five paternosters. After, remove the needle gently from the top part. If it happens that the cataract reascends, reduce it towards the lower angle, and when you have introduced the needle into the eye, do not draw it out unless the cataract be situated in the place described above; then gently extract the needle in the same way as you put it in, turning it about between the fingers. The needle being extracted, keep the eye closed and make the patient lie flat on a bed, keeping him in the dark with his eyes shut, so that he does not see the light or move for eight days, during which time put white of egg on twice a day and twice during the night."

Passing over four centuries, we come to an even more interesting description of the operation from the pen of Bartisch of Dresden: "The day being decided upon, on which the operation is to be performed, the doctor who is obliged to, or who wishes to do it, must abstain from wine for two days beforehand. The patient must also fast the same day, and must neither eat much nor little till an hour after the operation. Given the aforesaid conditions, try and procure a well-lighted room, in which the patient may have everything necessary for going to bed and remaining there, as he ought not to be taken to any place far off; the nearer to bed the better. Set thyself on a bench in the light and turn thy back to the window. The patient may be seated on a chair, a stool, or on a box, before thee and near to thee; in any case he is to be seated lower than thyself. His legs between thine and his hands on thy thighs. A servant stands behind to hold the patient's head. The servant should bend a little, so that the patient may rest his head against him (Fig. 1). When the patient is blind of one eye only, the other eye should be bandaged with a cloth and a pad so that he cannot see. Then take the instrument or the needle in one hand, so that the right hand will be for the left eye, and *vice versa*. With the other hand separate with great care the upper lid from the lower, using the thumb and the first finger, so that thou canst see how to direct the needle into the eye. When thou wishest to introduce the needle, the eye must be turned towards the light and looking straight at thee; also, I should make the patient turn his eye a little towards his nose, so that thou canst use the instrument better and that thou wilt not injure the small veins of the eye, but respect them. Direct the needle straight and with attention over the membrane called the conjunctiva, straight towards the pupil and uvea, at the distance of two blades of a knife from the membrane called cornea or from the grey that is in the eye. Hold the needle quite straight, hold it steady so that it will not deviate or slip. Hold the needle and press it, and turn it with the fingers in the eye with great gentleness, according to the instructions you may gather from the figure, which shows an eye in which the cataract has been taken away, while the other eye has not been touched (Fig. 2). Hold the needle firmly while turning it round, and be careful always to have the point towards the middle of the eye, that it almost touches the pupil and the uvea; and not to oscillate by any chance towards one side. When thou feelest that the needle has penetrated into the eye, that it almost touches the pupil and the uvea, and when thou hast proved to be really in the eye, hold the needle securely and move it, letting it slip backwards and forwards towards the pupil till thou art certain of being in the substance of the cataract, which thou canst easily be sure of by the movement of the cataract material. When thou hast remarked that, lower it carefully and gently and slowly, so as not to disturb the cataract; but try and free the matter entirely from the pupil and from the uvea with care, and keep it intact. Press the said matter with the needle under it, with the greatest care, and when thou perceivest that it is altogether free and loose, draw and direct the needle, with the matter behind it, upwards, and then pass it well downwards, behind the thin retina and the aranea of the eye; and take care that it remains there. . . . This is the recognised instruction, research, and indication of the means of operating, of pricking the cataract, or of the manner in which such an operation ought to be initiated and conducted. But no one ought to undertake such an operation unless he has learnt much and seen much, and unless he is fundamentally taught by intelligent doctors. Unless he is so, it is not well to operate. And it is not wise to trust to any of the brotherhood who happen to be dressed in velvet or silk, and who boast of being great oculists, and are capable of curing the blind from cataract. Certainly these can make holes in the eyes, but I do not know how they can succeed."

The knowledge which the Greeks and the Arabs possessed, before and after the dawn of the Christian era, on the subject of the pathology and treatment of cataract, appears to have been largely forgotten during the Middle Ages. It would seem that both couching and extraction fell into disuse, and that the surgical treatment of cataract was left for centuries in the hands of wandering charlatans, whose ways brought much discredit upon it. Towards the close of the seventeenth century, Pierre Brisseau, a doctor of Tournay, revived the operation, inventing a needle of his own for the purpose. His advocacy of the method aroused bitter controversy, but it was undoubtedly the best operation in the field until the famous French surgeon Daviel performed his first extraction in 1745, and thus sounded the death-knell of a procedure which had held the pride of place in European surgery for over seventeen centuries. It was, however, many years before couching was definitely abandoned in favour of extraction. Indeed, the author has recently had the privilege of discussing this subject with a distinguished surgeon, who can remember the time when depression was still a recognised method of operating in London. It is a great mistake to suppose that Daviel was the first to endeavour to extract a cataract, for both extraction and suction of cataracts have their roots far back in history. Indeed, Antyllus described his method of extraction at the close of the first century of the Christian era, and there are numerous other references to it in early literature. What Daviel did was to adopt a technique which gave a reasonable prospect of success.

The introduction of reclination, as opposed to depression, by Willburg in a Nuremberg thesis, dated 1785, gave a fresh lease of life to couching in its dying struggle with the operation which was destined to supersede it. England, France, Sweden, Germany, and other countries, joined vigorously in the discussion, and amongst the powerful advocates of couching were ranked Percival Pott and William Hay of London, Cusson of Montpellier, and Scarpa of Pavia, whilst Benjamin Bell practised both couching and extraction. The admirable treatise by James Ware on cataract (1812) was all but a death-blow for Celsus's operation. The newer procedure was then well in the ascendant, and only needed time to completely strangle its rival. Notwithstanding this, it was left to Mackenzie, so late as 1854 (fourth edition), to give the most complete and interesting description of couching to be found in literature. He distinguishes sharply between the operations of depression and reclination. In depression, the lens is pushed directly below the level of the pupil, being made to follow the curvature of the eye, to sweep over the corpus ciliare, until it comes to rest on the lower curve of the eyeball, with its anterior surface directed forward and downward (Fig. 3). In reclination, the lens is made to turn over towards the bottom

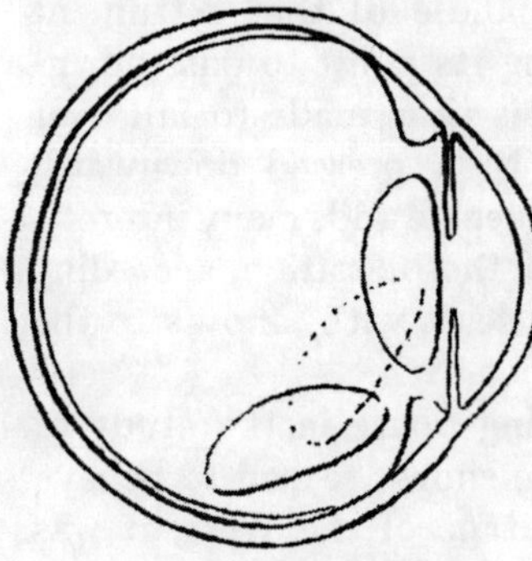

FIG. 3.—DEPRESSION.

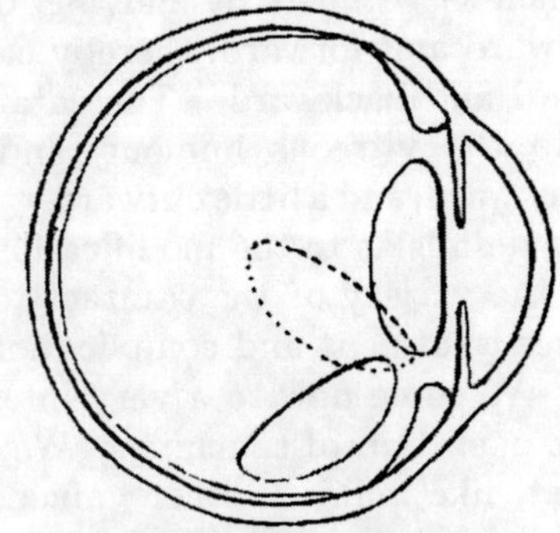

FIG. 4.—RECLINATION.

The above two figures illustrate the path taken by the cataract during the operation. (Mackenzie.)

of the vitreous chamber in such a way that what was formerly its anterior surface now comes to look upward, and what was its upper edge is turned to the rear. The whole lens is swung backward as if on a hinge, composed of the lower fibres of its suspensory ligament, which still remain unbroken (Fig. 4). He divides the operation of couching into four stages, in only the last of which reclination differs from depression. These are: (1) the pushing of a special needle (Fig. 5) through the coats

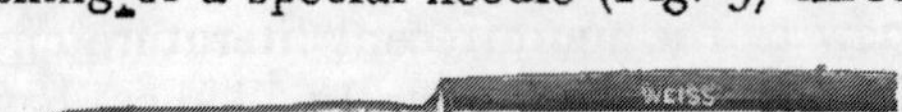

FIG. 5.

of the eye at a distance of $\frac{1}{6}$ inch behind the temporal edge of the cornea, and to a depth of $\frac{1}{6}$ inch; (2) the laceration of the posterior capsule of the lens by vertical movements of the point of the needle, to prepare an aperture for the passage of the lens; (3) the passing of the needle into the anterior chamber around the edge of the lens, and the laceration of the anterior capsule by vertical strokes; (4*a*) to depress the lens, the point of the needle is carried over its upper edge, and the handle is raised a little above the horizontal, thereby correspondingly lowering the point, which forces the cataract downward out of sight behind the pupil: the needle is then withdrawn by rotation; (4*b*) to effect reclination, the needle-point is raised not more than $\frac{1}{10}$ inch above the transverse diameter of the lens: its concave surface is pressed against the cataract, which is reclined by moving the handle of the instrument upward and forward, thereby causing its point to pass downward and backward. The cataract is thus made to fall over into the vitreous humour, and is then pressed downward, backward, and a little outward. Mackenzie adds many interesting details as to the modifications of the operation, according to the variety of the cataract to be dealt with, and as to the after-treatment and complications met with.

We come now to a very interesting phase in the study of the operation of couching. We have shown reason to believe that, like many another valued heritage of the West, it was brought there originally by Wise Men of the East. For more than eighteen centuries it remained a treasured possession of surgery, only to yield its ground before the fierce competition of a method better able to survive the stern test of experience. Slowly but surely its decadence banished it from modern scientific European literature, and then, strangely enough, the advent of Listerism fanned the dying flame of interest in the method; but this time in the East, and not in the West. From the East it had sprung to find a home in the West, and in the East, at the hand of Western surgeons, its last, and by no means least, interesting chapter is in the course of being written. A review of the more recent literature on the subject will establish this contention, and will show how large a share the officers of the Indian Medical Service have taken in the settlement of a question which, apart from its scientific value, has important social and even political bearings.

After a brief visit to India, Hirschberg, in 1894, published an article on couching, in the course of which he spoke favourably of the results of the operation. He was, unfortunately, handicapped by his ignorance of the natives of India and of their ways and customs, with the result that his views on the subject are of comparatively little interest to us. In the following year Captain H. E. Drake-Brockman described the operation of couching as explained to him by one of its Indian exponents. The latter pierced the sclerotic with a small lancet in the lower outer quadrant close to the cornea, and then introduced a copper needle; "a series of motions of the hand are made from the position on first introduction of the needle to a point corresponding to it in the upper section of the outer diameter of the eyeball." The depression of the lens appears to have taken place next, but the description is throughout somewhat vague. Presumably the operation was the same as that described by Ekambaram, but the coucher does not seem to have been able to make the steps of the procedure as clear as that surgeon has done.

Henry Power, in the *British Medical Journal* (October, 1901), entered a plea for the occasional performance of the operation of depression in cases of cataract. His experience went far enough back to enable him to remember the time, not only when he had seen surgeons of repute employ this method, but when he had himself imitated the example thus set. His own practice had been to attack the cataract, via the sclerotic, through the posterior capsule. He framed a number of indications which to his mind justified the occasional performance of couching. It is safe to say that very few of these would be seriously entertained by surgeons to-day. The most interesting point he made was in connection with Himly, in whose work, published in 1843, the statement occurred that "severe inflammation rarely followed reclination, and when it did it often cleared up without leaving any bad consequences." A doubt as to the reliability of Himly's statements is suggested by his claim that he had only two failures in fifty cases, one of these not being attributable to the operation. This is so much at variance with the experience of others as to make one sceptical about accepting any of his assertions without some reservation.

The next paper of value that we come to is by Maynard (1903). In this he analysed sixty-three cases of couching, which he had met with in Indian practice, and recorded the anatomical examination by Parsons of a couched eye sent home for the purpose. The same year saw the appearance of a paper by Albertotti of Medina, in which that writer somewhat fanatically and unconvincingly advocated a return to couching, with the use of a corneal puncture and with the employment of special instruments for the purpose. A year later he was followed along the same lines by Basso of Genoa, whilst Quartillera published a paper whose recommendations were very similar to those made by Henry Power. In 1905, Major Henry Smith of Jullundur, in a very outspoken article in the *Indian Medical Gazette*, expressed the opinion "that lens couching at the present time is an operation which should not be practised outside the ranks of charlatans," and added that "it is no easy matter to completely dislocate the lens, and in my observation the partial dislocation is more frequent than the complete in the hands of adepts of the art." In reply to this paper, Maynard reaffirmed his belief that couching is "justifiable under certain conditions." The editor of the *Indian Medical Gazette* invited further discussion of the subject, and in accordance with this request the writer published his statistics based on 125 cases of couching, carefully recorded on printed schedules. In the course of that paper he voiced his strong opposition to the adoption of the Indian operation, or of any modification of it, in the hands of surgeons who enjoy the unique opportunity of obtaining manipulative skill granted to those who work in India. A former pupil of his, Dr. Ekambaram, studied the ways of the Indian coucher at first-hand, and gave the results of his experience in one of the most valuable contributions to the subject yet made. This was in 1910. Two years later the writer was able to review the statistics of 550 consecutive cases of couching, all of which had been carefully noted. Still more cases accumulated before he left India, and by the kindness of Major Kirkpatrick, the total under review has now reached 780.

The examination by J. H. Parsons of a couched eye has already been mentioned. In 1913, A. C. Hudson sectioned and described a similar specimen sent him from India by the writer. The only previous published records of the same kind are from the pen of E. Treacher Collins, and refer to four specimens of couched eyes in the Museum of the Royal London Ophthalmic Hospital. Major H. Kirkpatrick has recently examined several more cases in Madras, and has kindly communicated some of the more interesting of his findings to the writer. Communications, that have been made from time to time before meetings of ophthalmologists, show that British surgeons of the first rank are still in favour of performing couching under certain special conditions. A marked instance of this is to be found in the discussion which took place before the Ophthalmological Society of the United Kingdom on February 8, 1906, following the presentation of a case by Holmes Spicer. On that occasion Rockliffe and Treacher Collins stated that, like Spicer, they had performed the operation in exceptional cases, and Devereux Marshall and G. W. Roll accorded it a modified support under such conditions. The writer has also learnt from personal communications that other leading surgeons have taken a similar line. There for the present we must leave the history of this operation, whose origin is lost in the dim mists of antiquity, and whose chequered career forms one of the most interesting pages in the literature of medicine.

BIBLIOGRAPHY

ALBERTOTTI, GIUSEPPE: Benevenuti Grassi, de oculis eorumque ægritudinibus (réédition de l'incunable de Ferrare, 1498); Paris, 1897.

ALBERTOTTI, GIUSEPPE: Depression of Cataract, La Clinica Oculistica, June, 1903.

AMERICAN ENCYCLOPÆDIA and Dictionary of Ophthalmology, Casey Wood; Chicago, 1916.

BASSO: La Clinica Oculistica, January, 1904.

BLAND-SUTTON, SIR JOHN: On an Apocryphal Miracle, Middlesex Hospital Journal, vol. xx., No. 1.

BRISSEAU: Traité de la Cataracte et du Glaucome; Tournay, 1706.

CELSUS, A. CORNELIUS: Of Medicine, trans. by James Grieve; printed by D. Wilson and T. Durham, Strand, London, 1756.

COLLINS, E. TREACHER: R.L.O.H. Rep., 1893, vol. xiii., p. 308.

CUSSON, M. P.: Remarques sur la Cataracte, à l'Académie des Sciences de Montpellier, 1779.

DRAKE-BROCKMAN, Surg.-Capt. H. E.: The Indian Oculist and his Equipment, Trans. of the O.S. of the U.K., vol. xv., 1895.

DRAKE-BROCKMAN, Lieut.-Col. E. F.: The Indian Oculist and his Equipment, Trans. of the O.S. of the U.K., vol. xv., 1895.

EKAMBARAM, R.: Couchers and their Methods, Ind. Med. Gaz., 1910.

ELLIOT, R. H.: Couching of the Lens, Ind. Med. Gaz., August, 1906.

ELLIOT, R. H.: The Operation of Couching as practised in Southern India: a Review of 550 Cases, Proc. of S. Ind. Branch of B.M.A., 1912, and Ophthalmic Review, vol. xxxi., 1912.

ENCYCLOPÆDIA BRITANNICA.

GALEN: De partib. art. med.

HAY-WILLIAMS: Practical Observations on Surgery; London, 1803.

HIRSCHBERG: Centralblatt für Praktische Augenheilkunde, February 1, 1894.

Hirschberg: Centralblatt für Praktische Augenheilkunde, 1908, vol. xxxii., p. 2.

Histoire de la Médecine, par Kurt Sprengel, trad. par A. J. L. Jourdan; Paris, 1815.

Histoire de l'Ophthalmologie à l'École de Montpellier, par H. Truc et P. Pansier; Paris, A. Moloine, 1907.

Hudson, H. C.: R.L.O.H. Rep., vol. xviii., part ii.

Mackenzie, W.: On the Diseases of the Eye, 4th edit., London, 1854.

Maynard, F. P.: Ophthalmic Review, April, 1903.

Maynard, F. P.: Ind. Med. Gaz., May, 1905.

Paulus Ægineta, vol. ii., Sydenham Society, 1845-46.

Pott, Percival: Remarks on Cataract.

Power, H.: Depression in Cases of Cataract, Brit. Med. Journ., October, 1901.

Quartillera, Castilley: Arch. de Oftal. Hispano-Americanos, October, 1904.

Smith, H.: Cataract Couching, Ind. Med. Gaz., May, 1905; and Trans. of the O.S. of the U.K., 1904, p. 264.

Ware, James: The Cataract and Gutta Serena, 3rd edit., London, 1812.

Wilkinson, Miss K. E.: The Manuscripts of Naples and the Vatican, etc., trans. from Albertotti, Ind. Med. Gaz., October, 1904.

CHAPTER II

THE TECHNIQUE OF THE OPERATION

THE writer has never seen a native coucher at work, and consequently all his information on the subject has had to be gathered from those who have been more fortunate than himself in this respect. There would appear to be two distinct modes of operating, which for convenience' sake may be spoken of as the anterior and the posterior, using the terms relatively to the plane of the ciliary body and iris (Figs. 6 and 7). We shall take them in turn.

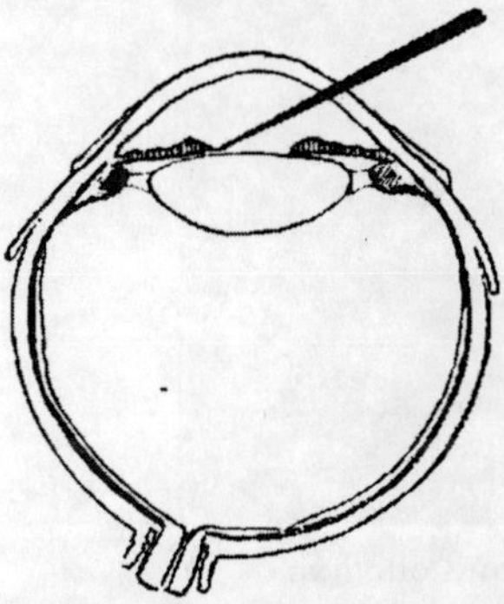

FIG. 6.—ANTERIOR OPERATION.

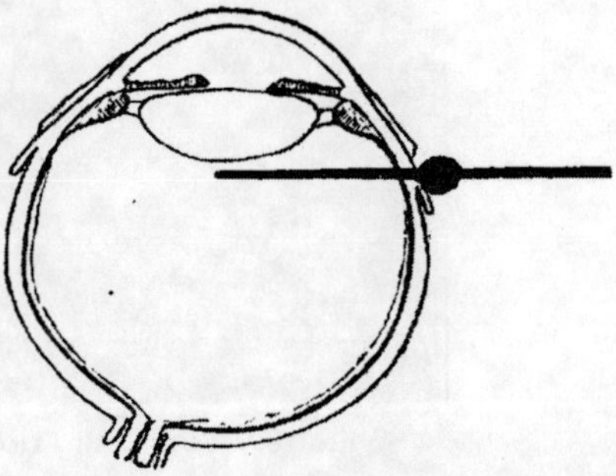

FIG. 7.—POSTERIOR OPERATION.

The Anterior Operation.—The patient and operator sit facing each other in a good light; both squat on their hams in accordance with the immemorial custom of the East (Fig. 8). The patient is frequently, if not usually, told that no operation is to be performed, and that it is merely a question of putting medicine into the eye. He is directed to look downward, and the coucher raises the upper lid with one hand whilst in the other he conceals either a needle or a sharp thorn. It is said that the long needle-like thorn of the babul-tree is usually selected for the purpose. Many of the patients have mentioned that their heads were steadied by a friend from behind. In the majority of cases, at least, it would appear that no form of local anæsthesia is attempted. The operators appear to rely largely on manual dexterity, and to aim at completing the procedure in a minimum of time. The needle or thorn is thrust suddenly through the cornea, and on through the pupil or iris, into or on to the periphery of the lens. The next movement, which appears to follow the first so rapidly as practically to melt into it, is that of depression or re-

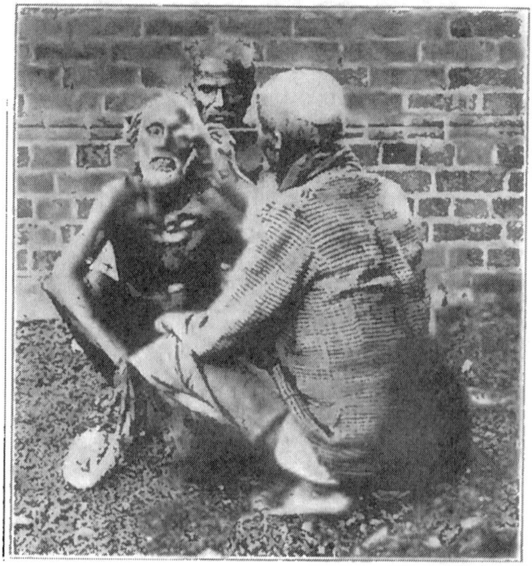

FIG. 8.—THE OPERATION OF COUCHING.

clination. In this, the spot where the cornea grasps the shaft of the needle serves as a fulcrum. The operator raises his end of the instrument, and the opposite one, which lies either on the surface of the lens or imbedded in it, is consequently depressed, thus carrying the cataract with it downwards, or downwards and backwards, and so clearing the pupil. In the course of speaking to a very large number of patients thus operated on, it has struck the writer as most remarkable that they made as little complaint as they usually did of the pain inflicted on them during the operation. They described the sensation of a sudden prick, but it was obvious that they had no acute recollection of agonising suffering. This point is emphasised by the fact that in nearly every case the operator tested his patient's vision immediately after the operation by holding up fingers, coloured cloths, necklaces, or other common objects, for triumphant identification. Very great stress is laid on this part of the ritual, and the onlookers are not allowed to lose sight of the wonderful results achieved by the operation. There seems reason to believe that an effort is made to enter the point of the instrument through the pupil, and to pass it between the iris and the lens. This cannot fail to be a difficult thing to do, as is evidenced by the frequency with which we were able to discover scars in the iris, which had obviously resulted from tears at the time of the operation. The point of perforation of the cornea could frequently be discovered, especially if a loupe were used for the purpose. The relative positions of the scars in the cornea and iris were frequently of great value to us from the diagnostic point of view. The eye is bandaged for at least twenty-four hours. By the end of that time the operator has frequently placed a safe distance between himself and his patients of the day before, and is seeking fresh dupes in another village.

The Posterior Operation.—Much that has been written on the preceding method applies with equal force to this. It is, however, possible to describe the technique much more accurately, as it has been carefully studied at first-hand by Dr. Ekambaram, who for many years worked under the writer in the Government Ophthalmic Hospital, Madras. His original description of the method will well repay a careful perusal. He speaks of the operators as being ambidextrous and very skilful. Their surgical equipment (Fig. 9) for the operation consists of a small lancet-shaped knife, guarded to within a few millimetres of its tip by a roll of cotton-wool, wrapped round it for the purpose, and of a copper probe 4 inches long and about 1½ mm. in diameter. A cotton thread twisted round this probe at a spot 12 mm. from its point serves the same purpose as the stop in the Bowman's needle. From the point to this stop the instrument is triangular in section. The patient is directed to look well towards the nose, and the surgeon then gently marks out the selected spot by pressing with his thumbnail on the conjunctiva covering the sclera, about 8 mm. out from the cornea, and about 2 mm. below the horizontal meridian. In some cases the operator steadies the eye by firm digital pressure exerted through the partly everted lower lid. He next takes his lancet in his hand, and it will be observed from the illustration (Fig. 9) that it might easily pass for a roll of cotton-wool; this, indeed, is what the patient is led to believe it really is. To heighten such an impression, the point is covered with a sandalwood paste, prepared beforehand *coram publico*, with a good deal of ostentation. The patient is informed that this "cataract-cleansing drug is about to be applied to the eye," and under cover of the suggestion the operator plunges the lancet through the tunic of the globe at the spot already

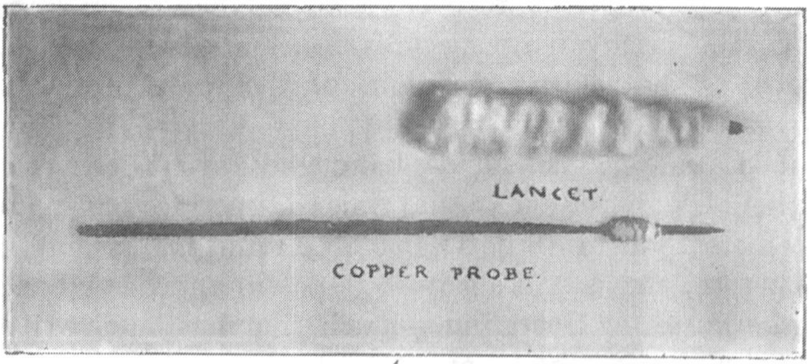

FIG. 9.—INSTRUMENTS USED IN COUCHING.

selected. The alarm thus occasioned is allayed by the assurance that the "medicinal application" is over. The copper probe is next produced, and is inserted through the wound up to its stop, being held between the thumb and two fingers; a circular movement is given to its point, the stop resting against the puncture, and serving as a pivot for the movement. According to Ekambaram, the object is to tear through the suspensory ligament from behind. Immediately following this step, a downward stroke of the point is made in order to depress the now loosened lens. Ekambaram graphically describes the care taken by these operators to impress, alike on the patient and on the friends, the magical effects of the procedure. The former is shown a number of objects, and is bidden to name them in turn, and to state their colour. The crowning point is reached when the surgeon removes a thread from his garment, and the patient not merely recognizes it as such, but triumphantly tells its hue. The Western ophthalmic surgeon, with his wide incision and his anxiety for the safety of the vitreous, can never savour such dramatic moments as these. They carry us back to the descriptions of the early Christian miracles, with all the mental and spiritual associations, which enwrap such stories as those of Bartimæus, and of the pools of Siloam and Bethesda. Alas that life's "hereafters" should so often be fraught with disillusionment, disappointment, and suffering! Palestine and its storied past rise before us as we read how the vaidyan called for a white cloth and for water, how he dipped the cloth in the fluid and washed out the sufferer's eye therewith, how he made a paste and smeared it over the skin around the brow, how he closed the eye with "clean white linen," and then sent the erstwhile blind man rejoicing away. Over the abyss of nearly twenty centuries, the East stretches out her unfaltering hand to the past of the nearer East, whilst the West looks on in wonder, not unmixed with admiration, for a spirit which the corroding passage of time seems unable either to fret or to change.

There is a step of the procedure which has been purposely left to the last, as its interest is psychologic, and not surgical. It is common to both methods of operation. I refer to the anointing of the eye with the blood of a freshly killed fowl. It is a measure in which superstition, cunning, self-preservation, and greed, overwhelm and mask a faint and feeble therapeutic design. The sacrificial element is present, and a hazy idea that the death of the votive bird may turn evil from the patient looms in the background. Next comes the need to mask the shedding of the patient's blood, since he is often told that no operation is to be performed, but that a mere "medicinal application" is to be made; the blood of the outraged bird covers the guilt of the vaidyan's falsehood. Largest of all towers the fact that the curry-pot even of a worker of surgical marvels needs constant replenishing, and that fowl is an excellent substitute for mutton on such occasions. Lastly, these men seem to believe that the coagulation of the fowl's blood helps to close the puncture. In view of the dirty condition of the instruments which they introduce into the interior of the eye, this last factor may practically be neglected.

CHAPTER III

THE INDIAN COUCHER AND HIS HABITS

THE coucher goes by different names in different parts of India. In Bengal and in the United and Central Provinces he is known as the " suttya " or " mal," and in the Punjab as the " rawal." Ekambaram, who came into intimate contact with these men in the Madras Presidency, always describes them as " vaidyans," the term signifying surgeons. In the north they are Hindus, of the Kayasth caste, a class well known for its astuteness and educational qualifications. Drake-Brockman states that in the north Mahomedan couchers are rare, whilst in the Southern Presidency it appears to be the exception to find a Hindu doing such work. Like every other occupation, couching in India is hereditary, the principles of the craft being handed down from father to son by word of mouth and by practical instruction. It has been stated that there is no literature on the subject. This, however, would appear to be a mistake, for Ekambaram learnt that there are " some old texts written on palmyra leaves laying down the method." A literal translation of one of these runs: " Removing the lancet after making a puncture, insert the copper probe; and holding it with three fingers, depress the lens with the three-sided edge."

By tradition and ancestral habit, the coucher is a wanderer on the face of the earth, and like a gipsy he carries his wares, such as they are, to the very doors of the people's homes; but it is probable that in each of the large provinces of India these men have a headquarters of their own. This in the Madras Presidency is known as " Kannadiputhur," which signifies the " village of eye operations." During part of the year these men are agriculturists and fishermen; but when the dry season robs them of their occupations, they wander forth to practise the art, with which their ancestors have been identified from time immemorial. They do not, however, confine themselves to eye operations, but practise as well a crude form of general surgery. Like many other disciples of Æsculapius, their fee is a very elastic one, and, in common with other artists, they learn to know both the smiles and the frowns of fortune. Luxury rarely comes their way, whilst hardship and toil are their constant lot. Their spare evening hours are filled in with such arduous and monotonous occupations as net-weaving; and full many a night they go hungry to sleep, with the sun-baked earth for their only bed.

All, who have seen them at work, agree that their methods are dirty and septic to a degree, and the oft-expressed wonder has ever been, not that their results are so bad, but that they are ever good. Their surgical equipment is carried in a bag or in a box, which would be considered dirty alongside of the tool-chest or work-basket of any English artisan. The filth alike of their clothes, their hands, and their person, stagger description from a surgical point of view. The exact patterns of the instruments used vary in different parts of India, and so also do some of the couchers' customs. Allusion has already been made to the slaughter of a fowl and the use of its blood in Southern India. This is readily understood, as the Mahomedan couchers are flesh-eaters. In the north, where these experts are Hindus, the fowl plays no part, but a very subtle form of deception is described by Drake-Brockman. Each suttiah carries in a little bag a store of pieces of dried membrane. One of these is dropped into water before the operation commences, and is produced at the psychologic moment as evidence that the Indian surgeon can, and does, remove the cataract from the eye, just as much as his Western brother. This tribute to our science is as subtle as it is nefarious. The pieces carried are of various tints, in order that the colour of the cataract, as seen before operation, may be matched as closely as possible.

Right through the ages the shadow of charlatanism has lain over the operation of couching. We are told that it did so in Alexandria and in Rome at the dawn of the Christian era, and from that time up to the present we find numerous traces of it in literature. Not the least interesting of such comes from the Dark Ages, and, despite its pathos, has a distinctly amusing side. The operator and his assistant took the patient alone into a darkened room; a candle was lighted and kept carefully behind the victim's back by one of the knaves, while the other in front asked if he could see the flame. A sham operation was then performed, and the process was again repeated, but this time with the light in front; naturally the blind man could now see it, and, on being assured that "the change" was due to what had been done, his gratitude was likely to rise to the production of the necessary fee. If it did so, the impostors speedily made off. It seems hard to believe that even the Dark Ages were dark enough for so transparent a trick to be tried often in one town.

In a recent personal communication, Dr. Ekambaram has very kindly furnished the writer with some additional information, as new as it is interesting. He divides the Indian couchers, with whom he has come into contact, into two classes, the Mahomedan couchers of the south, whose work we mainly meet with in Madras, and the Punjabis (people of the Punjab) from the north. The same method of operation is adopted by both, but there would appear to be a great difference between the status and the attainments of the two classes. The Mahomedans are much the lower type; their practice is confined to the villages through which they roam, and they very rarely visit big towns. Their length of stay is limited to one or two days, and they make haste to escape soon after having performed an operation, "for fear of being clubbed for their stupid action." They do not use any form of anæsthetic. On the other hand, the Punjabi couchers are described as intelligent, respectable, decently clad men, who confine their work to the towns, and stay in each place four or five months, amassing considerable wealth thereby. Before couching, they drop into the eye a fine yellow powder, which Ekambaram believes to be stained cocaine. They were, however, extremely secretive on this subject, and refused to part with even a grain of the drug at any price he could offer. Its efficiency is testified to by the fact that the patients remained absolutely quiet and collected during the whole of the operation. The cases are kept under observation for from a week to a month after operation, putting in a daily attendance. Their results are much better than those obtained by the Mahomedans.

Some of the fees they obtain are relatively very large. An idea of their social status may be gathered from the fact that carriages are sent for them by their better-class patients; but, in Ekambaram's opinion, the aristocracy of Indian intelligence is learning to keep aloof from these men, owing to the influence of the Western surgeons, whose method of extraction is steadily establishing itself in the esteem of the people at large. He gives credit to the Punjabis for a more efficient technique of operation than that practised by the Mahomedans.

In this connection it is interesting to record some of the opinions of Western surgeons, who have come in contact with the work of these northern men. Captain H. E. Drake-Brockman had nothing too bad to say of them, and his uncle Lieut.-Colonel E. F. Drake-Brockman (formerly of the Madras Eye Hospital), in presenting his nephew's paper before the Ophthalmological Society of the United Kingdom, estimated the coucher's successes at not more than 10 per cent. Lieut.-Colonel Henry Smith went so far as to declare that even the best cases, if followed long enough, ended in absolute blindness. Lieut.-Colonel F. P. Maynard formed a much less unfavourable estimate of the coucher's results (46 per cent. of successes). The writer's own statistics will be given later. Not the least interesting of Drake-Brockman's contributions to the subject is his statement that vaccinators and compounders in the pay of the Indian Government are not infrequently couchers in disguise. The full significance of this observation can only be appreciated by one who knows the East intimately. Scientifically, Western medicine is educating the Indian medical man out into the light from pagan depths of darkness. Even to-day there are those of them who practise Eastern and Western medicine side by side. It would seem strange to a British surgeon to learn that it is possible for a medical man (whose qualifications, from an educational point of view, compare favourably with those of our home Universities) to lay stress before his patients on the right quarter of the moon, and on the correct aspect of the ground, for the gathering of a particular drug; yet the writer has known this happen, and that, too, in the case of a medical man who held an important scientific appointment under Government. The very fact of a man holding a post under the British Rāj would add to his prestige and increase the confidence of the people in him. That such an one should advocate and practise couching would cause no surprise to his own people, whose faith in methods based on tradition is firmly founded. Some idea of the complexity and confusion of the Indian mind today may be gathered from a knowledge of the strange blend of dissimilar lines of thought in those who have adopted Christianity. There are many such who keep a foot in both camps, in a way that would have been thought impossible by anyone who had not been brought into intimate contact with such people. Under these circumstances, it is hardly strange that the same kind of thing should be found in evidence in other lines of life; and yet it is no time to blame these men. Their need—I speak now from the scientific standpoint—is for "more light." We ourselves retain to-day the taint of superstitions that come down from our witch-burning ancestors. Shall we not, then, be lenient to those who have never had our advantages? As we flood India with the daylight of true scientific knowledge, the vermin of ignorance and superstition will scurry away to hide. That the coucher believes in himself is indisputable; that he resents the invasion of our Western operation is easily understood; and that he must disappear, washed out by the advancing flood of better methods, is as certain as the fate of the furrows left on the sand by last night's tide. Meanwhile he has stopped a gap and filled a place in the life of a nation, and it behoves us, in our estimate of him, to remember that the highest earthly honour ever awarded was given to a woman whom the world despised and blamed, in the immortal words: "She hath done what she could."

It has been said of these men that they have no diagnostic powers, and it is quite certain that they sometimes couch the lens in cases of optic atrophy, of glaucoma, and of certain other diseases, in which such a step is useless and worse. It is fair to add that the number of cases of this kind which the writer saw was not large. This observation is the more significant, since he was keenly on the lookout for any instances of the kind, and that, too, during many years of Indian experience in an exceptionally large cataract practice. Ekambaram speaks of a case of operable cataract in which he had dilated the pupil, and on which he (purely experimentally, and with no intention of allowing it to be done) asked couchers if they would operate. As soon as they found the pupil was motionless and dilated, they declined to undertake any operation. He comments favourably on the acumen they thus displayed.

A word may not be out of place on the subject of the covering of the head of the patient and surgeon with a cloth, as adopted by some few couchers during the operation. Such a procedure is, from the point of view of lost light, a handicap to the operator, but it has, from his way of looking at it, certain advantages. It shuts the patient off from the distractions of his surroundings, which are otherwise very public; it hides the actual operative procedure from prying eyes; and it conceals the facial and other evidence of pain. The greatest factor of all, in an Eastern land, is the air of mystery with which it shrouds the proceeding. The element of "jadu" (magic) so introduced is paramount in its psychologic interest.

CHAPTER IV

STATISTICAL

In the *Indian Medical Gazette* of August, 1906, the writer published a review of 125 cases of couching of the lens by Indian vaidyans. On March 13, 1912, the total had swollen to 550, and an analysis of all the cases was conducted on the same lines as those followed in the earlier communication. Subsequent to this, Major H. Kirkpatrick, the succeeding Superintendent of the Madras Eye Hospital, analysed 350 cases of the Mahomedan operation (the first 120 of which overlapped the series already dealt with by the writer), and in forwarding them made the comment that "these statistics are remarkably similar to those of your series." In view of the consistency of the results obtained and of the large figures dealt with it seems safe to assume that reliable deductions can now be drawn.

The main headings of these statistics will next be taken up. Before commencing to do so, it is of special interest to note that the methods observed by Colonel Drake-Brockman in other parts of India tally closely with those described by Ekambaram in Southern India. This is the more readily understood when we remember that many of the operators in the South of India come from the north. This observation puts our cases on all fours with those published from other parts of India.

It is perhaps difficult to form an accurate opinion as to how far the figures before us represent the best results attained by the coucher. His apologists might urge that only his failures would come to English hospitals. On the other hand, there can be little doubt that quite a considerable number of eyes are lost, after couching, from panophthalmitis and from shrinkage of the eye following iridocyclitis. Patients in such conditions will often stay away from hospital owing to their very hopelessness; and even if they do resort to English treatment, they will stoutly deny that their eyes have been interfered with. Thus in both ways the records of such failures are lost, making the net result appear better than it really is. In collecting our statistics, we were constantly on the lookout for *all* cases of couched lens, and have notes of a large number of patients who did not come to hospital for the eye in which reclination had been performed.

Considerable interest attaches to the study of the column showing the periods that elapsed between the Mahomedan operation and the date at which the patient came under observation. Only 6·82 per cent. were seen within the first month, and but 17·88 per cent. within the first six months. The following six months added only 5·65 per cent. The great mass of the eyes had been operated on from one to ten years previous to being seen. This in itself would indicate that the cases, from which our observations were made, were drawn from the mass of the people rather than from the coucher's failures alone.

An argument in support of the reliability of our figures may be drawn from the extraordinarily widespread opinion, amongst both European and Indian practitioners, that the vaidyans' results are appalling. The writer had the opportunity of talking on the subject with a large number of men who practised in the parts where couching was rifest, and their testimony was unanimous. Ekambaram, who has already been freely quoted, has made these men's methods a special study, and, impressed by the wholesale destruction of eyes he had witnessed, made the request that the matter should be brought to the notice of Government through the Surgeon-General, which was accordingly done. Apropos of the figures now under discussion, Colonel Drake-Brockman wrote: "I have seen quite enough to convince me of the truth of Major Elliot's statement, and that his percentage of actual loss of eyes from this cause alone is by no means exaggerated." Major Smith has given his experience of the disastrous results of couching, and has gone so far as to say that even the best cases, if followed long enough, end in absolute blindness. With this last observation we cannot wholly agree, nor do our statistics in the south bear out his opinion that "partial dislocation is more frequent than the complete dislocation in the hands of adepts in the art." He is satisfied that a great majority of cases go bad immediately, either from suppuration or from iridocyclitis, and that a large proportion of the remainder are but imperfectly couched. Other surgeons, too, have testified to the disastrous nature of the vaidyans' results.

Only 4·94 per cent. of the total number of cases lie below the age of 36, and nearly 69 per cent. lie between the ages of 40 and 60. This is in accordance with what we know of senile cataract in India. Of the fourteen cases which show an age of 30 or below, eight may be excluded as having probably given their ages too low; one was lost by suppuration after couching, and no deduction can be made as to the condition before operation; in two it seems probable that the cataract was secondary to syphilitic iritis: they were two eyes of different persons; in one patient the operation failed on both sides: the eyes were congenitally imperfect, and in addition iritis was present as a complication in one of them. In the sixth the operator evidently burst the capsule and let out its semi-fluid contents; but the nucleus remained *in situ* and blocked the pupil. It is obvious that couching is an extremely unsuitable operation for this class of case; it requires for its easy performance a firm lenticular mass, but as will be seen when we come to discuss the morbid anatomy of the subject, it is quite possible to dislocate one of these fluid lenses intact. There is at least a presumption that in such cases the posterior operation has been performed, though, in view of the toughness of the capsules of not a few Morgagnian cataracts, one cannot say with certainty in all such cases that the anterior operation has not been done.

No table is more interesting than that which gives the state of vision when the patients came under observation. In only 10·59 per cent. was the vision $\frac{1}{3}$ and upward. In another 11·05 per cent. the vision was $\frac{1}{4}$ to $\frac{1}{10}$, in 9·64 per cent. it was $\frac{1}{10}$ to $\frac{1}{30}$, and in 7·05 per cent. it was a finger-count at 2 feet or less. The figures given refer in each case to the vision corrected with lenses. If every case that got a vision of $\frac{1}{10}$ and upward be considered a success, the coucher can claim 21·64 per cent. Again, if anything from $\frac{1}{10}$ vision to the ability to count fingers close to the face be counted as partial success, the figure for this class is 16·69 per cent. This is very much more liberal treatment than would be accorded to the cataract statistics of any modern surgeon.

A further light is thrown on the above figures by a study of the table showing the duration of vision after couching. Of the 45 successful cases, 23 of them, or more than 50 per cent., had been couched less than two years before; 9 more had been couched between two and three years, and 11 from three to ten years. In two this detail was unmarked. The great preponderance of short histories in the cases of successful operation is significant.

Against the vaidyans' figures we may place the statistics of the Madras Hospital, even so long ago as 1903, and before a rigid system of antisepsis had been introduced. Recoveries numbered 96 per cent., poor results 2 per cent., and failures 2 per cent. These figures would indicate that the coucher was losing 60 per cent. more eyes than the hospital did even then. If the vast number of eyes submitted to couching be taken into account, this 60 per cent. of avoidable loss totals up to a staggering figure. Nor must we disregard the fact that, even amongst the successes, the average vision obtained is greatly in favour of the Western surgeon.

The table showing the causes of failure will repay a careful study. The figure for iritis and iridocyclitis comes to 35·76 per cent. of the *total* number of cases; glaucoma accounts for 11·05 per cent., imperfect dislocation of the lens for 8·94 per cent., retinal detachment for 3·53 per cent., optic atrophy (including one case of optic neuritis supervening as a septic complication of the operation) for 2·59 per cent., retinitis pigmentosa and retinitis punctata albescens for 0·49 per cent., retinochoroiditis for 1·41 per cent., vitreous opacities (admittedly a very vague term) for 1·18 per cent., and failure due to operation on a congenitally imperfect eye for 0·23 per cent.; 3·53 per cent. are, unfortunately, unaccounted for owing to deficiencies in the notes.

In the great majority of cases ruined by iridocyclitis the inflammation made its appearance within a few days after operation; but there were instances in which this complication was delayed for a long period. Our notes show three cases in which it came on from one and a half to three years after operation, one case after seven years, and one after ten years. There are also a few doubtful cases in which a history of three or four months of useful vision preceded the inflammatory attack. In one case at least, sympathetic ophthalmia would appear to have destroyed the other eye two years after operation.

Similarly, it was found in most cases of glaucoma that the access of high tension came on within a few days of operation. There were six exceptions to this rule, three commencing from two to ten months after the couching, one five years, one six years, and one fourteen years after. From a clinical point of view, the cause of the onset of glaucoma in these cases is obscure. Many of them appear to be associated with iridocyclitis, but we must leave this matter for the present. We shall have occasion to deal with it much more fully under the heading of pathology.

Imperfect dislocation of the lens accounted for failure in 8·94 per cent. of all cases operated on. In such cases the suspensory ligament appeared to have been incompletely torn, with the result that the lens swung, as it were, on a hinge. Sometimes this hinge lies above, and the cataract falls quite out of the line of sight when the patient is recumbent, but flaps back to block the pupil when the erect attitude is assumed. In other cases, even when the hinge is laterally placed, the same thing may happen, but much more rarely.

From a clinical point of view, detachment of the retina figures in only 3·53 per cent. of the total cases; but it is unlikely that this represents the true figure. In a number of instances an ophthalmoscopic examination was quite impossible, either because the pupil was blocked, or because no fundus reflex could be obtained. Our pathological material has shown that in many such cases the retina was totally detached, whereas, in arriving at the figure above given, we were dealing only with those instances in which the diagnosis was established by the aid of the ophthalmoscope.

Ten of the cases in which failure was ascribed to optic atrophy showed no improvement in vision after operation. Their histories indicate that the atrophic condition was present before operation, and there seems to be a fair presumption that the coucher mistook the condition for cataract, or at least failed to recognise its true nature. In one case acute optic neuritis appears to have supervened as a septic complication of the operation. This throws an interesting light on those pathological specimens in which a cone of exudate is to be seen passing from an inflamed optic nerve to the ciliary body.

In six cases there was evidence of choroido-retinitis with secondary optic atrophy. Four of them showed no improvement after operation, whilst two were improved thereby; subsequently even these two lost their vision by the progress of the retinitis. In the four cases the retinitic condition was evidently antecedent to the operation, and was either mistaken for cataract or at least was not recognised. It is impossible to say positively, from the history of the other two, whether it existed prior to operation, but it possibly did.

In one case of retinitis pigmentosa, in one of retinitis punctata albescens, and in eleven of glaucoma, the vaidyan appears to have mistaken the condition present for cataract. At least, the vision was not bettered even temporarily by the operation in any of these patients.

Of the five cases shown under vitreous opacities, three were obviously due to the inflammation of the uveal tract posterior to the iris; two others were due to hæmorrhage into the vitreous. Many more cases would undoubtedly have shown vitreous opacities had the pupils been patent. Moreover, our pathological data show that not a few of the cases in which the fundus reflex was absent presented dense exudates into the vitreous cavity. This subject will be dealt with at length under pathology. The genesis of hæmorrhage into the vitreous is obvious, and it is more than probable that if all the cases were seen at an early stage the figure for this complication would be much higher.

From the foregoing notes, it is clear that the native coucher undertakes a certain number of what we should recognise as inoperable cases. It is possible that in many of them a secondary cataract is present; but it is clear that his diagnostic powers are low. He is a standing menace to the safety of the public.

It has from time to time been suggested that the presence of the lens in the vitreous chamber brings about retinal changes. The author is not, however, aware of any reliable evidence either ophthalmoscopic or pathological to support this view As far as possible, all cases seen in Madras were submitted to ophthalmoscopic examination, whether the couching had resulted in success or failure. We were unable to discover any characteristic change which could be attributed to the couching. A large percentage of the fundi examined appeared to be absolutely normal. The most frequent departure from normal was an undue distinctness of the choroidal vessels, which was evidently due to the absorption of the pigment of the pigmentary layer of the retina. It is probably this phenomenon which has misled some into the belief that couching is followed by changes in the retina allied to those in retinitis pigmentosa *sine* pigmento. This absorption of retinal pigment is, however, well known to occur in other conditions, as, for instance, in high myopia; moreover, in the case of couched eyes, it is not accompanied by the changes in the disc and vessels characteristic of retinitis pigmentosa, or by the equally characteristic night blindness. In searching for the explanation of this phenomenon, four solutions at once present themselves for consideration: (1) It might be, as has been suggested, a result of couching; (2) it might be due to the alterations in the refractive conditions under which the fundus is seen; (3) it might be a physiological abnormality; and (4) it might be an accompaniment of, and a direct result of pathological changes in the eye accompanying the development of cataract. The third suggestion is thrown out by our experience of normal native eyes. An important light has been thrown on the whole question by the observation that a similar change is found in quite a number of eyes which have been submitted to cataract extraction. This disposes of the first idea, that the presence of the lens in the vitreous would account for the phenomenon. Neither experience nor theory support the view that an alteration in refraction is responsible for the appearance. We are thus narrowed down to the conclusion that the pigmentary change is an accompaniment of the development of cataract in a certain percentage of eyes, and is independent of the method of operation resorted to for the relief of that condition.

In this connection, two interesting observations deserve record, as they possibly throw an important sidelight on the question at issue: (1) Lenses extracted in India differ from those met with in European practice, in the amount of colouring matter they contain. A very large percentage of them are stained with pigment, which is frequently of a deep tint. Many of them are dark brown, and a few are almost black. (2) Cyanopsia is of extraordinarily frequent occurrence as a sequela during convalescence after cataract extraction in Madras. Over 50 per cent. of the patients complain of it, whilst only 2·8 per cent. suffer from erythropsia, and 1·2 per cent. from yellow or green vision.

We thus find two very striking differences between Western and Eastern cataract experience, and there is, to say the least of it, a strong suggestion that the phenomena are closely connected with each other—in other words, that the cyanopsia is a result of the retina becoming tired out for the perception of yellow by long exposure to a tropical light filtering through a brown or yellow lens. There is also a strong presumption that the coloration of the lenses is due to a migration of pigment, which takes place during the development of cataract in the East, a migration which is directed from the pigmentary layer of the retina, and probably from other parts as well, towards and into the developing cataracts. If the above hypothesis is correct, we might assume that the retina is more likely to be functionally affected in an adverse sense when deprived of the protection ordinarily afforded by its pigmentary layer. In order to test this, the author some years ago made a systematic examination of a large number of eyes from which cataracts had recently been removed, with the object of ascertaining whether cyanopsia was complained of, principally or only, in those cases in which the choroidal vessels were seen to stand out with unusual distinctness under ophthalmoscopic examination. The depth of discoloration of the lenses was at the same time noted in each case. The results obtained appear to favour the views we have above enunciated, but they were not sufficiently conclusive to justify the formation of a decisive opinion. It must be remembered that, whilst a tinge of colour runs through most of the cataractous lenses removed in the East, there are very wide variations, not only in the depth of the pigmentation, but also in the actual coloration present. Some of them are yellow, some reddish-brown, some almost coal black, with every intermediate shade between. It is possible that our investigations failed for want of competent assistance with the spectroscopic analysis of the lenses. An interesting field for research is here presented. That deep-seated metabolic changes accompany the development of a cataract has been shown by J. Burdon Cooper, and it seems not unlikely that the apparent prevalence of lenticular opacities in tropical countries may be closely bound up with the metabolic changes we have described. It is probable that the retinal pigment layer is not the only source of the deep discoloration of the lenses met with by surgeons in India. A point in favour of the argument we have been elaborating is that some years ago McHardy published the analysis by MacMunn of the spectrum of the pigment obtained from a black cataract. This was found to be quite distinct from blood-pigment, and to be allied to the cell-pigment, which gives coloration to ectodermal structures in animals (Trans. of the O.S. of the U.K., 1882).

To collect the 780 cases now under review has taken over twelve years, and the writer is deeply indebted to Major Kirkpatrick for his great generosity in allowing his 230 cases, the later ones of the series, to be made use of in this paper. Throughout all these years one definite purpose has been kept in the forefront—viz., to ascertain the real value of lens couching. After making every possible allowance for the vaidyan, the fact remains that he is a standing menace to society, and that he should be suppressed. His methods are crude, filthy, and dangerous; his results are so appalling that anyone unacquainted with the ignorance and credulity of the Indian ryot would think it impossible for him to continue to exist. His impudent lying includes not merely a grossly exaggerated statement of his own successes, but extends to the most barefaced falsehoods as to the nature of the results obtained in European hospitals. It may be permissible to quote one instance—unfortunately, far from a solitary one in Madras experience. Some years ago a peasant, who had had a cataract removed in the Government Ophthalmic Hospital, and whose recollections of his treatment there were most kindly, returned for operation on the second eye. On the steps of a temple, within a hundred yards from our operating theatre, this man, who had travelled several hundred miles for aid, was induced, by a tissue of impudent lies, to sit down and submit to couching. A few days later he presented himself at the out-patient room with panophthalmitis. There is no branch of ophthalmic disease and treatment in India which so profoundly impresses the Western surgeon's imagination as this one. Remember that cataract strikes a man down in his maturity, at a period of his life when he has begun to reap the benefits of his earlier years of toilsome industry. His pay and his home expenses are both alike at their maximum. He is treading the higher rungs of the official or business ladder, and is endeavouring to afford his children the best education in his power. Few pictures are more pitiful than that of such a man passing hopefully down an avenue of credulity and ignorance to a fate to which death itself is often preferred, the horror of a great and lifelong darkness. On the other hand, Government, the protector of the poor, stands by powerless to interfere, and supinely watches this catastrophic waste of human energy. The cords that bind the individuals are woven a million-fold together to tie the hands of the rulers more securely still. Every civilized nation of today recognises it as a first principle, that it is its duty to protect its people from avoidable harm, and that to deal with preventable blindness is one of its primary duties. That men and women, who ought to be burden-bearers, should be thrown instead as a burden on their relatives or on the State, is a social evil of no small magnitude. One does not presume to blame either the State or the people. It would obviously be idle and wrong to do so. The plain indication is to arouse the medical conscience of the country, to start men thinking of the evils which are so rife in the land; and so to introduce a ferment, as it were, into the medical mind of India, and then to leave it to do its work. It is not suggested that the country is ripe for legislation on the subject. The people are not ready for it. There are, however, two distinct avenues along which an advance may safely be made—viz., (1) the systematic dissemination of knowledge through Government agencies amongst the people; (2) the improvement of ophthalmic medical education. A movement in these two directions is already on foot, and in time it will bear much fruit.

CHAPTER V

THE PATHOLOGICAL ANATOMY OF COUCHED EYES

BEING THE HUNTERIAN LECTURES DELIVERED BEFORE THE ROYAL COLLEGE OF SURGEONS OF ENGLAND ON FEBRUARY 19 AND 21, 1917

THE material at our disposal consists of 54 *globes*, the great majority of which were removed in the Madras Ophthalmic Hospital in the period from 1911 to 1915, though some are of much older date. They were placed in 5 per cent. formalin immediately on removal, and were subsequently frozen and bisected. In a number of instances one half of the eye was submitted to microscopic examination after suitable sectioning. Each of the half-globes and a number of microscopic specimens have been photographed for purposes of illustration. It will be convenient to classify our observations under a number of separate headings.

The Various Directions in which Dislocation of the Lens is found to have taken place.

Before considering this subject in the light of the pathological specimens before us, it is necessary to make certain preliminary statements:

1. Inasmuch as all our material is derived from blinded eyes, it is obvious that we are dealing with the coucher's failures alone, and are excluding his successes. In a very large percentage of the latter the lens is seen, during life, to be floating freely in the vitreous, apparently untrammelled by adhesions.

2. The position in which we find the lens on bisection of the eyeball is not necessarily that into which it was thrust at the time of operation, for the changes which occur in the eye

as a result of inflammatory action may profoundly alter the position into which the lens was originally forced by the coucher. Nor must we forget that in those globes, in which the cataract is not tightly tethered by adhesions, gravity plays a part.

Having thus cleared the ground, we may start with the statement that, though the lens may be displaced in any direction within the sclero-corneal coat, backward dislocations are by far the most common, whilst forward ones were only found 4 times in the whole series of 54 globes. None the less, each of these latter cases possesses considerable interest.

Forward Dislocations.—(1) In No. 8 * the couching instrument passed through the limbus, and the track of the wound can be plainly followed in microscopic sections. The ciliary body was pushed bodily away from the sclera, and the lens nucleus was forcibly thrust into the space formed by this cyclodialysis (Pl. II., Fig. 10); it is to be seen imbedded in a mass of inflammatory exudate, whilst its capsule, with some of the cortex, lies in the normal situation.

(2) In No. 44 the capsule and the nucleus of a Morgagnian cataract are seen floating in the vitreous chamber (Pl. II., Fig. 11). During life the nucleus frequently passed backwards and forwards between the aqueous and vitreous cavities. The same phenomenon, though rare, has been observed in other couched eyes.

(3) No. 61 is probably an instance of the same kind of thing having happened at an earlier period (Pl. II., Fig. 12). Now, however, the small dark Morgagnian nucleus is seen fixed in the lower part of the anterior chamber, into which it doubtless gravitated by its own weight, and there set up inflammatory mischief, which led to its adhesion to the surrounding parts, and to its becoming fixed *in situ* by the formation of organising exudate.

(4) In No. 108 the only evidence of lens material present was the capsule of a Morgagnian cataract, which lay impacted in the lower part of the anterior chamber (Pl. II., Fig. 13). On

* The whole series of specimens has been presented to the Royal College of Surgeons of England. The present chapter forms a descriptive catalogue of the most instructive of them. The original Madras numbers within the bottles have been retained, and are here quoted for ready reference.

PLATE II

FIG. 10: SPECIMEN NO. 8, WHOLE-SECTION.—The lens can be seen dislocated between the ciliary body and the sclera; the pectinate ligament had been ruptured at the operation.

FIG. 11: SPECIMEN NO. 44.—The small Morgagnian nucleus lies in the anterior part of the vitreous chamber; it passed freely between this and the aqueous chambers, sometimes appearing in the one, and sometimes in the other. The scar of the operation wound can be seen in the lower part of the illustration, close to the ciliary body. Notice the folds into which the detached retina has been dragged by the shrinking inflammatory exudate. A tongue, consisting of the posterior surface of the iris, was stripped back at the time of operation, and can be seen attached posteriorly to the front of the hyaloid body.

FIG. 12: SPECIMEN NO. 61.—A small dark Morgagnian nucleus lies impacted in the lower angle of the anterior chamber, which is largely filled by a flocculent coagulated exudate. Notice the coagulated subretinal exudate, and the cyst in the outer wall of the lower part of the retina.

FIG. 13: SPECIMEN NO. 108.—The capsule of a Morgagnian lens lies impacted in the angle of the anterior chamber; it had contracted no adhesions. The vitreous body is represented by a fine cone of exudate, which stretched forward from its apex at the optic nerve to a broad base at the ora serrata.

FIG. 14: SPECIMEN NO. 50.—A large Morgagnian cataract floated free in the vitreous chamber. The retina is extensively detached.

FIG. 15: SPECIMEN NO. 136.—A large hard laminated lens lies lightly imprisoned in the inflammatory exudate which formed in the vitreous body. A long curved scar can be seen over the ora serrata at the temporal side of the specimen.

PLATE II.

FIG. 10 (No. 8).—Lens dislocated between cil. body and sclera.

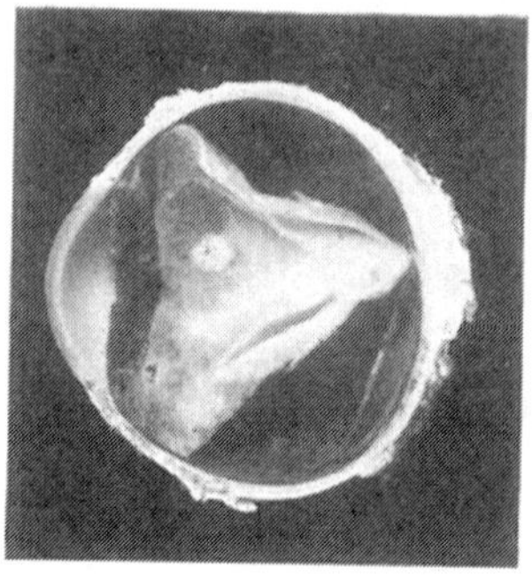

FIG. 11 (No. 44).—Left eye, lower half.

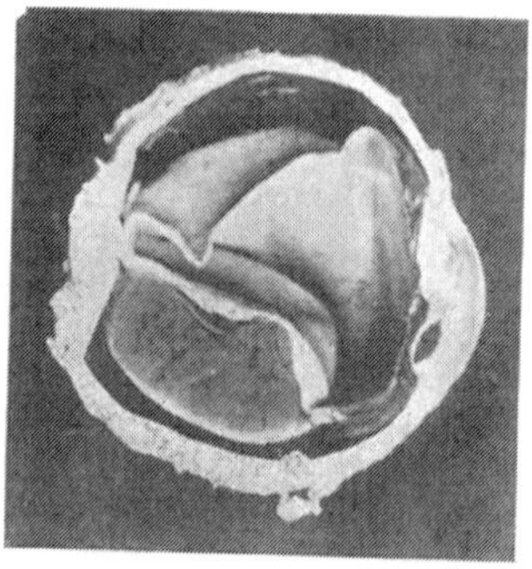

FIG. 12 (No. 61).—Left eye, temporal half.

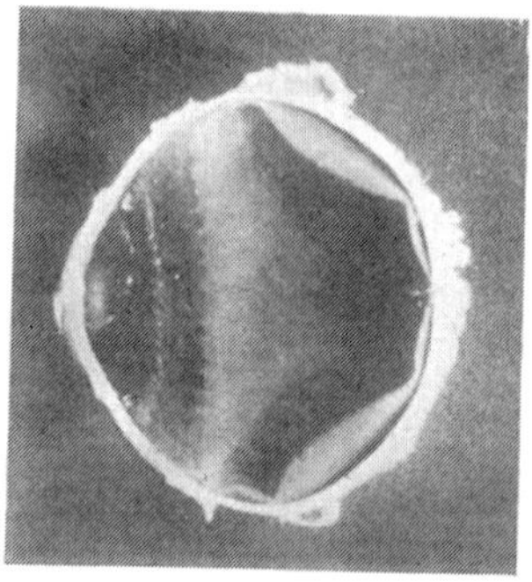

FIG. 13 (No. 108).—Right eye, nasal half.

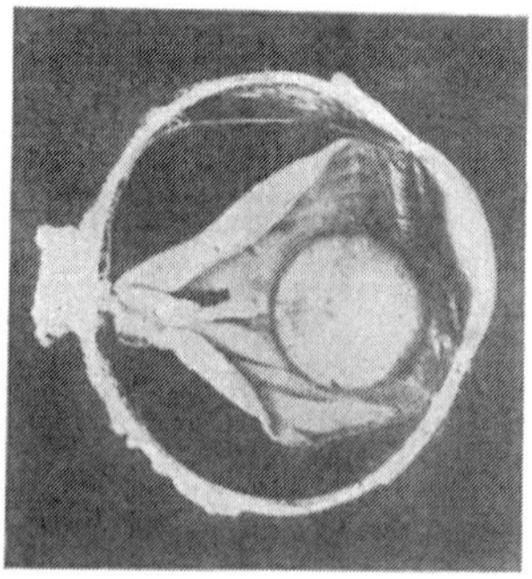

FIG. 14 (No. 50).—Right eye, lower half.

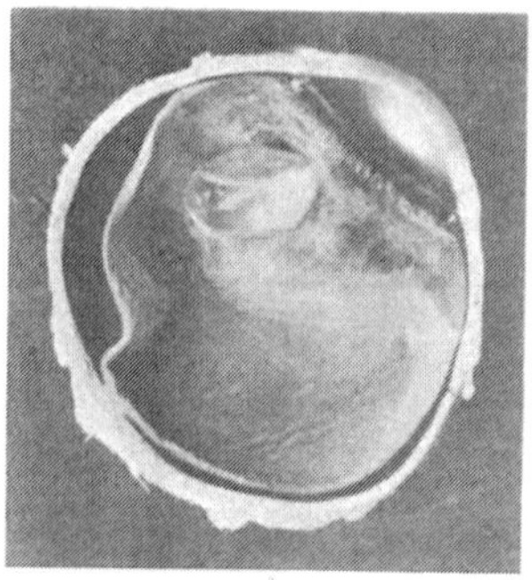

FIG. 15 (No. 136).—Left eye, upper half.

section, Morgagnian fluid escaped, and no trace of a nucleus could be detected. It is of interest to record that the writer has, on a number of occasions, operated on Morgagnian cataracts in which the lens nucleus had been reduced to the thickness of a lamellar disc, or in which no trace of a nucleus could be detected. In this case no adhesions had formed, and during the transit of the specimen to England the capsule fell from its position to the bottom of the bottle.

Backward Dislocations.—Dislocations backward are the rule, and very wide variations are found both in the completeness and in the direction of the displacement.

Those in which the *lenses*, or their nuclei, have been *completely dislocated into the vitreous, and there lie floating* more or less freely (Pl. II., Fig. 14), are 9 in number. In 7 of them the cataracts were Morgagnian, and in the 2 others there was a bulky nucleus with a thin covering of stiff cortex. In 7 the tension of the globe was high; in 6 the retina was completely or nearly completely detached, and in 2 of them it was so much folded as to limit the movements of the lens.

From a consideration of the lenses found floating in the vitreous, we turn to that of those which were *entangled in a more or less consistent inflammatory exudate occupying the vitreous chamber* (Pl. II., Fig. 15). During life such lenses were reported to be fixed, or nearly so. In the specimens they are seen to be nested in a mass of exudate, which holds them imprisoned against the ciliary body and the back of the iris. Usually this exudate is limited in quantity and is confined to the anterior portion of the eye, and principally to the neighbourhood of the dislocated lens. More rarely it is very abundant, and occupies a large part or even the whole of the vitreous chamber (Pl. III., Fig. 16). We shall deal with this exudate more fully at a later stage; for the present it suffices to state that it is inflammatory in origin, and that it contains a large number of cells. Of the 6 cases which form this group, 3 were Morgagnian cataracts; 5 were certainly dislocated in their capsule, the sixth is hidden in such dense exudate that it cannot be clearly seen. It is desirable to make it clear that intermediate forms are found between this group and the previous one. In other words, there is no hard-and-fast line between the cases in which the lenses float freely in the vitreous and those in which they are, to a greater or less degree, tethered by the pathological thickening of the hyaloid body.

We have next to consider a group of 10 eyeballs, in each of which the dislocated *cataract was firmly fixed to the ciliary body and to the back of the iris by definitely organised fibrous tissue* (Pl. III., Fig. 17). These globes present certain well-marked features of some interest: (1) The percentage of Morgagnian cataract is much lower than that in the preceding groups, and corresponds closely with the normal frequency of this form of cataract in Indian practice. (2) The cataract was dislocated *in its capsule* in no less than 8 of the 10 cases. (3) The retina was totally detached in 2 and very extensively so in one; in every one of the remaining 7 this membrane showed the presence of white dots, apparently on its surface. (4) The time which had elapsed since operation in the cases falling under this group is remarkable. In one it is given as seven months; in 2 others there is no history; in the remaining 7 the duration was from two to twenty years, with an average of well over seven years. The association of the presence of white dots with these long histories is remarkable, and will be taken up in a later section.

No. 99 (Pl. III., Fig. 18) is a specimen of special interest for two reasons—viz., (1) the cataract is fixed to the globe unusually far back, being attached to the retina a little behind the equator of the eye; (2) the dislocation has taken place in an upward direction, and therefore against the action of gravity. From time to time we meet clinically with a couched lens whose suspensory ligament, though torn through over a wide circumference, has been spared at one part, which acts as a hinge. The loosened lens flaps backwards and forwards with the movements of the eye, at times obstructing the pupil, and at others being lost to sight. If the hinge is above, the cataract usually blocks the pupil when the head is erect; but one meets with cases in which the lens floats up out of the way unless the face is thrown forward into the horizontal plane; this is apparently due to a check-ligament action of the remaining suspensory fibres of the lens, acting on a lens which is very nearly of the same specific gravity as the vitreous in which it lies. Should inflammation be set up in such an eye and the lens become involved in the exudate, it

PLATE III

Fig. 16: Specimen No. 197.—The exudate into the vitreous cavity is abundant and opaque, concealing the dislocated cataract. (Time since operation, one month.)

Fig. 17: Specimen No. 37.—The lens is tied to the back of the iris and ciliary body by firm organised exudate, which is continuous with and part of the cone of inflammatory material representing the shrunken vitreous. Notice the advanced organisation evident in the apex of the cone near the optic nerve, also the white line apparently representing the hyaloid canal. Some large dots and many small ones are to be seen on the retina.

Fig. 18: Specimen No. 99.—A large lens in its capsule is dislocated upward and inward, and is adherent to the retina by inflammatory bands. The retina shows very numerous white dots. There is a tendency to equatorial scleral staphyloma.

Fig. 19: Specimen No. 171.—The retina is totally detached and rolled up tight; cysts both false and true are to be seen in it. The lens is imbedded in a mass of inflammatory exudate, matted to the iris and ciliary body in front, and to the retina behind; the ciliary body is detached. The coagulated subretinal exudate gives the specimen the appearance of a half-marble. The sclera is folded owing to the shrinking of the eyeball.

Fig. 20: Specimen No. 119.—From before backwards can be seen the iris, the remains of the lens capsule, and the thickened anterior layer of the hyaloid. The lens is dislocated backward between the second and third of these, and is wedging them apart. The retina is detached over nearly half the globe; this is in large part determined by the pull of the shrinking thickened anterior hyaloid layer.

Fig. 21: Specimen No. 46.—The hard dark nuclear cataract had been depressed; it lies in front of the unruptured anterior hyaloid membrane, and therefore outside the vitreous cavity.

PLATE III.

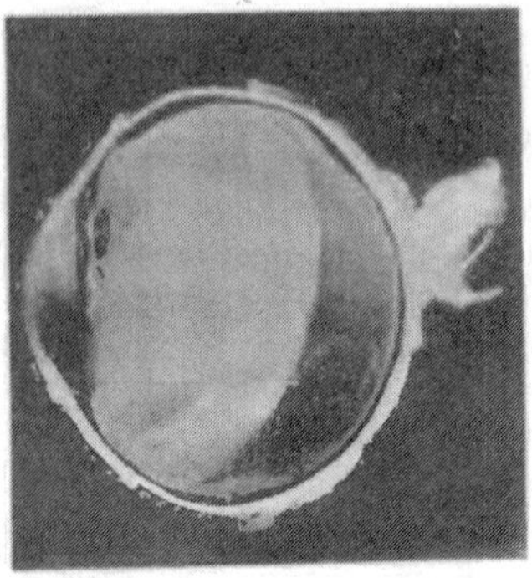

Fig. 16 (No. 197).—Left eye, lower half.

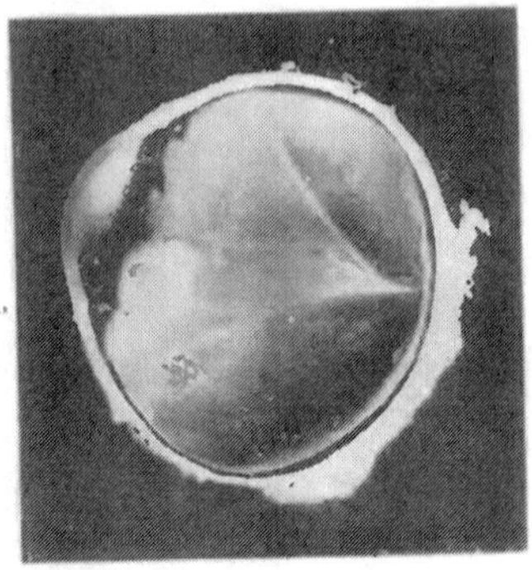

Fig. 17 (No. 37).—Left eye, lower half.

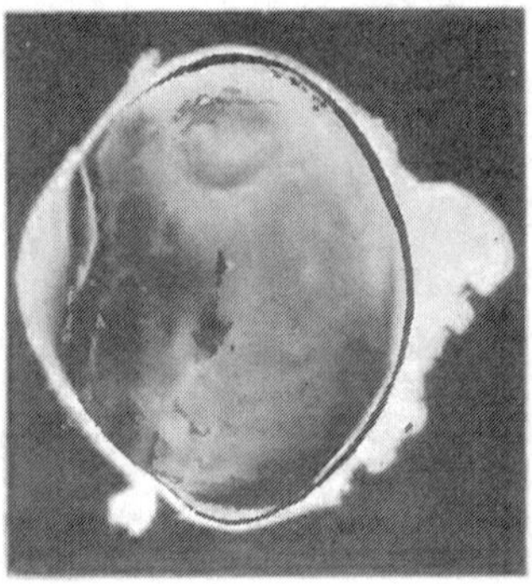

Fig. 18 (No. 99).—Left eye, upper half.

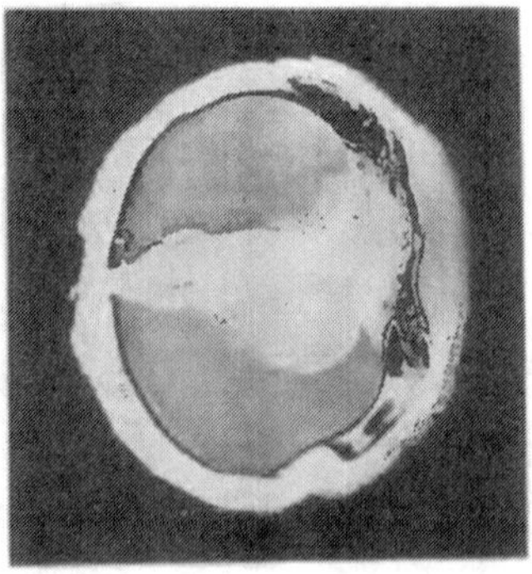

Fig. 19 (No. 171).—Left eye, upper half.

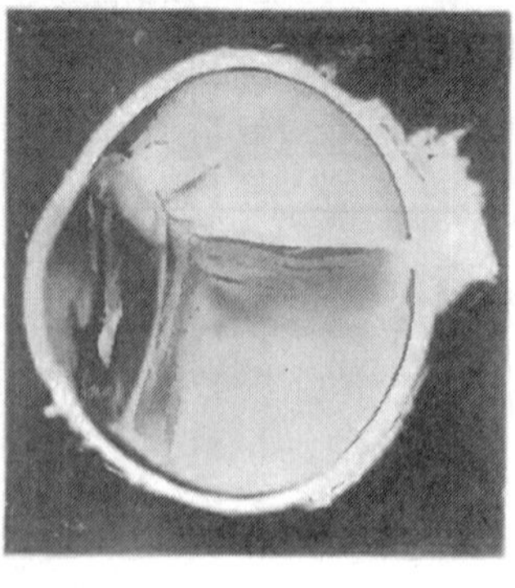

Fig. 20 (No. 119).—Right eye, upper half.

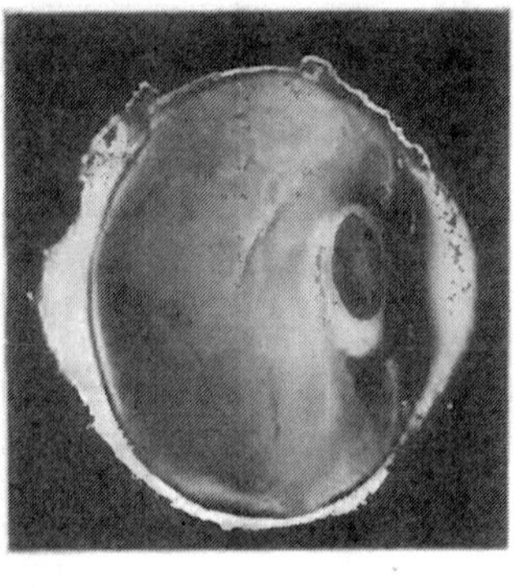

Fig. 21 (No. 46).—Left eye, lower half.

may become fixed, as in this case, in the upper segment of the globe.

When we come to speak of the changes found in the vitreous, we shall have occasion to refer to the frequency with which the hyaloid body is represented by a shrunken cone with its apex at the optic nerve and its base in the neighbourhood of the ora serrata. This form, which is well known to pathologists, is due to the anatomical attachments of the vitreous body, and to the fact that the latter undergoes shrinkage after being thickened and opacified by the presence of inflammatory exudate. In studying the present collection, one cannot fail to be struck with the fact that the exudate, which fixes, or helps to fix, the lens in its pathologic position, is one with, and part of, this cone-shaped new formation. Before leaving the consideration of this group, we must once again point out that no hard-and-fast line separates it from the preceding one, and that intermediate links between the two can easily be pointed to.

In 11 globes, *dislocated cataracts were found matted between the iris and ciliary body in front and the completely detached retina behind.* It is very difficult to say what the nature of the original cataracts was, since all that one can now find is a nucleus, usually rather dark-coloured, imbedded in a mass of inflammatory tissue (Pl. III., Fig. 19). These nuclei are undergoing steady reduction in bulk as the result of phagocytic action. In 7 of the 11, the lens remnants lie either within the complete capsule or in its near neighbourhood. The interior of the capsule is usually found to have been invaded by the mass of inflammatory and organising tissue which mats together all the structures (*i.e.*, the iris, the ciliary body, the remains of the lens, and the detached retina), and which occludes the angle of the anterior chamber. The completeness of the dislocation varies greatly. In some cases the lens is hardly moved from its usual position, and lies in front of the anterior hyaloid membrane, whilst in others it is displaced into the vitreous cavity. In one instance the detachment of the retina and the inflammatory changes are sharply limited to the lateral half of the eye towards which the cataract was dislocated, but this case belongs more to the next group than to the one we are now discussing.

There are three outstanding and very important features common to these cases: (1) In the great majority of them there is evidence that the operation was followed by severe iridocyclitis ; (2) 9 of the 11 were shrinking eyes with low tension; and (3) the time which had intervened between the couching and the enucleation was between one and two years in every case save one, in which it is probable that the furnished statement of three months was inaccurate. It will be noticed that the histories are much shorter than those in the previous group. This, together with the other two points mentioned, indicates that we have to deal with a condition widely different from that in any of the previous groups. Here the inflammatory process had been induced by a septic infection of the eyes of a decidedly more virulent character, though it fell short of that acme of infectivity, which leads in so many cases of the Indian operation to panophthalmitis and destruction of the globe within a few weeks.

We come next to a group of 5 cases, which have one feature in common—viz., that the cataract, though *dislocated backwards, lies distinctly in front of the anterior hyaloid membrane,* and therefore outside the vitreous cavity (Pl. III., Figs. 20 and 21). In 3 of them the solid parts of the lenses have been pushed back from their original position in such a way that they act like wedges, forcibly keeping the anterior hyaloid membrane in a plane posterior to that which it would normally occupy. Out of these 5 cataracts 4 were cortico-nuclear; the fifth was too much altered for it to be possible to state what its nature was. In certainly 4 out of the 5 moderately severe iridocyclitis had followed the couching, but the exudative process was a much less severe one than that which characterised the specimens of the previous group. The consequence was that there was no such matting of all the parts concerned as is there seen. In every case the detachment of the retina was complete or nearly so, but in not one was the lens enwrapped in its folds. This we may attribute to two causes: (1) a merely contributory one, that the vitreous cavity was not invaded; and (2) that the infection was less virulent, and the inflammation consequently less severe, than in the members of the previous group.

There is a small group of 3 cases in which the remains of the lens lie *in situ* in the periphery of the capsule, whilst the central portion has disappeared. These resemble the peripheral after-cataracts not infrequently seen following the extraction of a not fully mature lens.

In conclusion we have to mention 2 specimens in which the condition found was so unusual that it would scarcely have been possible to have anticipated its occurrence.

The first of these was one of the earliest globes sectioned. A Morgagnian lens, entire in its capsule, was found *thrust behind the retina.* It lay against the scleral coat close to the ciliary body; it had detached the retina over a large area in the neighbourhood of the ora serrata, and had led to a complete separation of it on that (the nasal) half of the eye. The edge of the detached retina had contracted adhesions to the front of the lens capsule, and was much puckered in that neighbourhood, doubtless as the result of cicatrisation.

The second specimen (Pl. IV., Fig. 22) shows many features in common with the last. The lens is entire in its capsule, and is almost certainly Morgagnian; the tear in the retina through which it was thrust has now cicatrised up, leaving a puckered scar. The retina is totally detached, and on section the cataract lay as far forward as the separation of that membrane would permit. The pupil was blocked by exudate, and atrophic scars in the iris showed that there had been extensive laceration of that membrane. The globe was removed a year after operation.

The sequence of events in these two cases was possibly as follows: The posterior operation may have been adopted and the incision placed far back; a wide tear in the retina resulted; the lens, completely separated from its attachments, was kept entire by the toughness of the Morgagnian capsule, whilst the fluidity of its contents made its insinuation through the retinal tear an easy matter. The fact that a case has recently been recorded in which, in a boy of seventeen, the lens spontaneously escaped through a 2 mm. trephine hole throws a sidelight on such cases as these.

Accidental Injuries to Other Structures than the Lens during Couching.

Though the primary object of the Indian cataract coucher is to depress the lens, he may accidentally injure any or all of the other structures of the eye. Evidence of such damage is obtained both clinically and pathologically.

The Cornea.—Opaque scars on the cornea are quite frequently seen in the out-patient room in eyes which have been subjected to the anterior operation, but are rendered invisible in formalin-mounted specimens owing to the opacification of the membrane. Other evidence of corneal injury is, however, available.

In No. 9 a corneal fistula is present, lying to the inner side of the centre of the eye (Pl. IV., Fig. 23). The lamellæ immediately surrounding it are largely replaced by connective tissue; the whole thickness of the membrane is markedly reduced, and the lining epithelium is irregular and vacuolated. The iris is very closely adherent to the back of the cornea near the fistula, but more loosely attached farther out. There has evidently been some ulceration of the cornea and the formation of a limited staphyloma, which burst at a later date, leaving the fistula now seen. It is probable that the point of fistulisation was determined by the use of a septic instrument at the time of operation, and that septic keratitis followed, leading to early perforation with entanglement of the iris. On the other hand, it is possible that the *enclavement* of the iris occurred as the instrument was withdrawn. In either case, the later sequence of events included a secondary rise in tension, the formation of a staphyloma, and a fresh perforation at the weakest point, resulting in the production of a permanent fistula.

In No. 45 the lens capsule is adherent to the back of the cornea, the iris being widely torn, and being probably also involved in the synechia (Pl. IV., Fig. 24). All that remains of the lens is a brown nucleus; the cataract was evidently Morgagnian. It is probable that, after the escape of the fluid it contained, the lax capsule prolapsed into the wound, either with the gush of fluid which accompanied the withdrawal of the instrument or at a later date.

In No. 116 it is the retina which is impacted in the corneal

PLATE IV

FIG. 22: SPECIMEN NO. 138.—A large Morgagnian cataract in its capsule lies dislocated behind the totally detached retina; the tear in the front part of the lower half of the retina, through which the lens was thrust, is now represented by a wide puckered scar.

FIG. 23: SPECIMEN NO. 9.—A whole-section showing a persistent fistula of the cornea.

FIG. 24: SPECIMEN NO. 45.—A brown nucleus dislocated downward in its capsule lies tightly adherent to the back of the iris and ciliary body; it is fixed there by organised exudate, the bands from which radiate out into the retina and are determining the detachment of that membrane. The iris is torn on the nasal side, and through the tear there passes a capsulo-corneal synechia.

FIG. 25: SPECIMEN NO. 116.—The retina is totally detached, and rolled up like a closed umbrella. There is a retino-corneal synechia. The lens has been reclined; it probably lay outside the vitreous cavity. The subretinal exudate, coagulated by preparation, gives the eyeball the appearance of a cut marble. During life the pressure of the lens, which had been wedged backward, thrust the retina and the parts adherent to it backward below, thus displacing the subretinal exudate there, and causing it to bulge in the upper half of the eyeball; this bulge effectually obliterated the upper part of the anterior chamber, whilst the direct pressure of the lens obliterated the chamber below.

FIG. 26: SPECIMEN NO. 306.—There is a pigmented scar running through the thickness of the sclera, just behind the level of the ciliary processes. The optic disc is deeply cupped, and the anterior chamber is very shallow.

FIG. 27: SPECIMEN NO. 306.—Low-power magnification of the previous specimen shows a persistent fistula running through the substance of the sclera; the ciliary body is impacted in its deeper part, and there is a filtering scar on its surface.

PLATE IV.

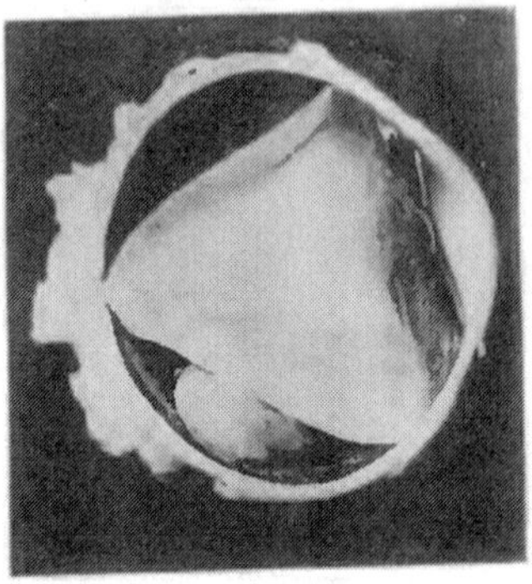

FIG. 22 (No. 138).—Right eye, lower half.

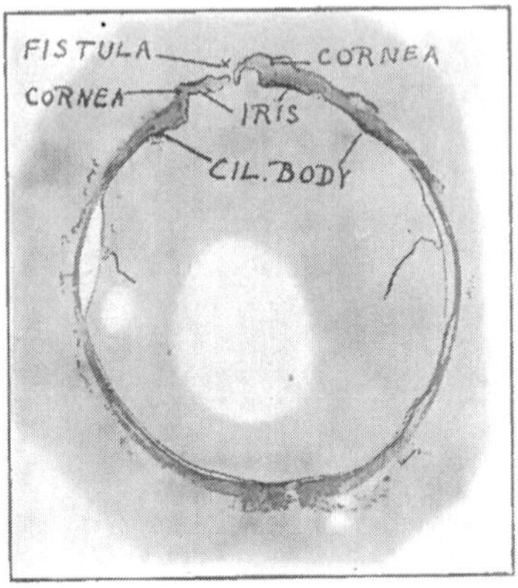

FIG. 23 (No. 9).—Left eye, whole section.

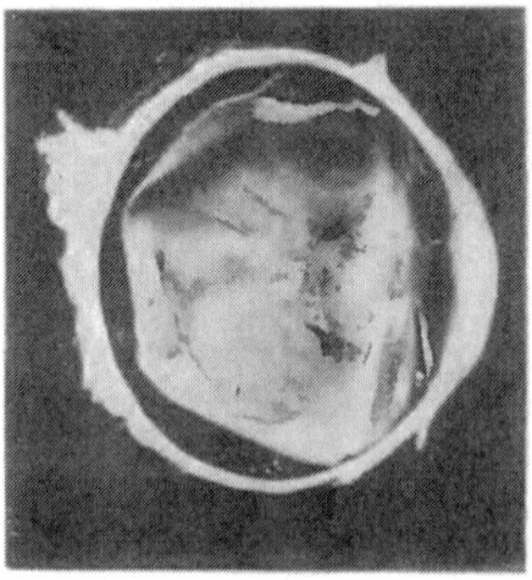

FIG. 24 (No. 45).—Right eye, lower half.

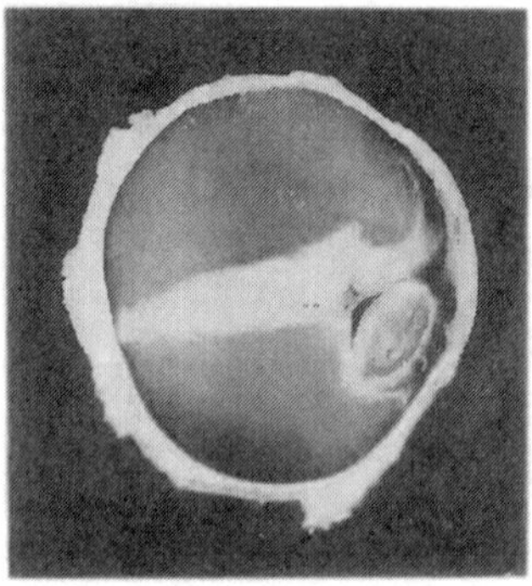

FIG. 25 (No. 116).—Right eye, nasal half.

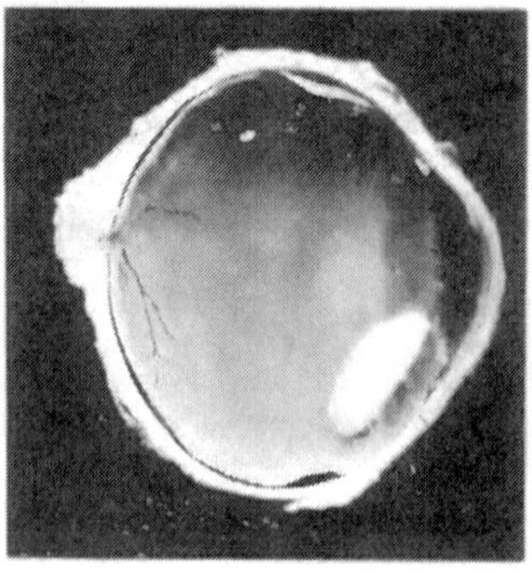

FIG. 26 (No. 306).—Left eye, upper half.

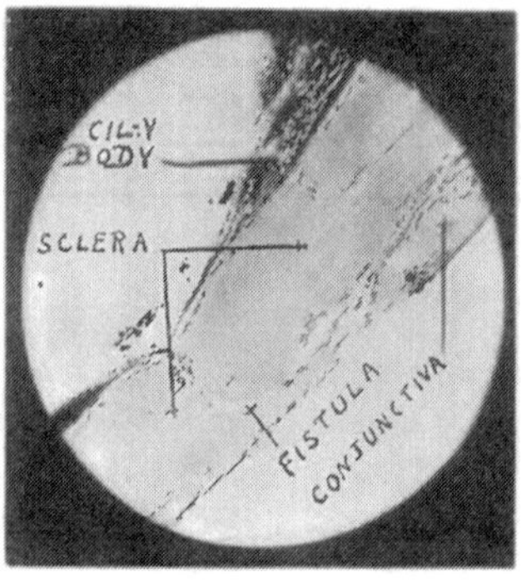

FIG. 27 (No. 306).—Microscopic section, low power.

wound (Pl. IV., Fig. 25). It seems likely that in this instance the sequence of events was as follows: A severe plastic inflammation resulted from the couching, and involved among other structures a capsular synechia, which had formed at the time of operation or soon after. The vitreous became heavily infected, and the consequent exudate became adherent on the one hand to the retina, which thereby underwent total detachment, and on the other to the capsule and its synechia. The progressive contraction of the scar-tissue then drew the retina into the wound. This would appear to be the most likely explanation, but it is not impossible, in dealing with such an operation as couching, that the retinal detachment was very extensive, and that the injury inflicted provided a path along which a direct prolapse of the retina may have occurred.

The Sclera.—A very large number of Indian cataract couchers perform the posterior operation, and therefore make their preliminary incision in the sclera outside the limbus. Dr. Ekambaram, who has watched these men at work, believes that they deliberately endeavour to avoid the ciliary body, and it also looks as if some of them purposely place their incision below the external rectus muscle. Like his Western confrère, the Indian surgeon does not always succeed in placing his incision just where he wishes to; this is not surprising, as many of these men work without any local anæsthetic, and not a few of their patients are nervous and unruly to the last degree. Moreover, it is more than probable that there are different opinions amongst couchers as to the best site for the preliminary cut. These considerations will serve to explain the variety of location of the scars, as found in the specimens before us; indeed, some such explanation is called for, since the cicatrices may be found as far forward as the limbus, and as far back as the equator of the globe; what is more, they may be seen in the present collection, not only in their common situation, on or near the horizontal meridian, but in any of the quadrants of the eye.

As a rule, the evidence of injury to the sclera is to be inferred from the interference with the parts beneath that coat, and such instances will be taken up when we come to consider the lesions of the ciliary body and choroid; but occasionally we have been fortunate enough to hit off the scleral scar either in the original division of the globe or during the course of sectioning of part of it for the purpose of microscopic examination.

In No. 306 the track of the original wound can be seen as a pigmented scar in the sclera immediately behind the line of the ciliary processes (Pl. IV., Fig. 26). Microscopic sections show—(1) that the pigmentation of the deeper part of the scar is due to the impaction of uveal tissue in its depth; (2) that there is a fistulous scar running right through the thickness of the sclera; and (3) that the subconjunctival tissue in the neighbourhood of the wound is permeated by large open spaces lined with endothelium (Pl. IV., Fig. 27). It is clear that a limited measure of filtration had been established, but this apparently proved insufficient to keep the tension of the eye from rising, as is shown by the deep glaucomatous cupping and by the obliteration of the anterior chamber.

No. 43 shows a scar a little farther back, in the neighbourhood of the ora serrata; but in this case the wound appears to have healed solidly. The pigment of the underlying uveal tissue shows a marked disturbance, whilst before the specimen was cut it was observed that the sclera was pigmented in the neighbourhood of the cicatrix.

In No. 8 the wound lay in the limbus, and the solidifying scar can be traced right through the thickness of the ocular tunic and down to the mass of inflammatory exudate which surrounds the dislocated lens, and fills the angle of the anterior chamber. Here, again, the pigment can be traced some distance up into the scar, in which the uveal tissue is distinctly entangled.

The Uveal Tract.—In quite a large number of couched eyes one can see, during life, evidence of past injury to the iris in the form of more or less extensive scars, many of which probably also involve the ciliary body. Moreover, in other cases, one can infer the presence of injury to the ciliary body and the choroid from the existence of pigmented cicatrices in the sclera. Anatomically, the present series of eyeballs affords additional information on this head. Iris scars are fairly common. In one case, already referred to, the coucher had effected a cyclodialysis; in 3 more the wounds lie across the front parts of the ciliary processes; in 6 they involved the region of the orbiculus ciliaris, and in one of these the scar lies as much on the choroid as it does on the ciliary body (Pl. II., Fig. 15); lastly, in 4 the wounds lie well behind the ciliary body, being placed in 2 of them just in front of the equator, and in 2 more well behind it. Taking them as a whole, the wounds tend to be grouped in the outer quadrant of the eye, above or below the horizontal meridian. It has already been pointed out that this is in accordance with Ekambaram's evidence as to the site of selection for the incision in the posterior operation. Far the best method of examining these scars is by transillumination with a bright light from behind. Some points of interest remain for consideration.

In No. 44 the wound lay behind the ciliary processes (Pl. II., Fig. 11), the instrument, most probably at its point, tore off a tongue-shaped process from the posterior surface of the iris, thus thinning that membrane over this area; the torn portion contracted an adhesion to the subjacent hyaloid membrane, which was itself infiltrated with inflammatory exudate; the appearance presented is curious and interesting.

In several of the globes scar-tissue radiates from the wound area into the surrounding tissues, and is then a strong contributory factor in the production of retinal detachment. In one globe (No. 130) two scars are to be seen, one of which was evidently placed too far back by mistake (Pl. V., Fig. 28); the eye also furnishes contributory evidence that things did not go well during the operation, for the iris is very widely lacerated. It seems probable that the patient was refractory or the surgeon unskilful. In any case, it is clear that the instrument was introduced a second time.

In No. 148 a caseating mass in the eyeball (Pl. V., Fig. 29), lying behind the equator, was found to contain a fragment of metal; the latter was most unfortunately lost at the time the section was cut, but it was presumably the tip of the couching instrument, and its presence, taken with the facts that the wound was placed very far back and that dislocation of the lens was not effected by the operation, would seem to indicate that the patient moved violently and that the operator failed in his purpose. The strong but strictly localised inflammation excited suggests that the metallic fragment was of copper, and this is in accordance with the known facts of the case, since the probes used by these men to displace the lens are made of that metal.

No. 72 is also a specimen of special interest. Here, too, the puncture lay behind the equator, and there seems to have been some difficulty in penetrating the choroidal and retinal coats, which were carried in front of the instrument, the result being a wide separation of these two tunics from their scleral bed (Pl. V., Fig. 30).

No. 297, removed six weeks after the operation, is an eyeball which had undergone panophthalmitis, and had burst through a point in the sclera on the horizontal meridian somewhere in front of the equator. It is probable that a septic wound of entrance determined the site of the bursting. The lecturer has seen suppurating globes in which the sclera at one point had completely sloughed, the intense inflammation present bearing witness to the violence of the infective process excited.

Uveitis.—The type of inflammation of the uvea found in these specimens was plastic, and was mostly confined to the iris and ciliary body. The intensity of the inflammation varied very greatly. In a number of specimens the evidence of inflammatory action was either absent or only to be detected on very careful examination. On the other hand, a large number of cases present themselves at Indian hospitals in which suppurative panophthalmitis has followed the operation of couching. In Madras such globes were eviscerated, as it was considered dangerous to enucleate them, and much interesting material has thus been lost. All the intermediate stages between the very slight and the very severe inflammations can be traced in the specimens before us. This is in accordance with what we should have expected in what was practically a series of inoculations of healthy globes with pathological materials, which varied enormously in their nature and in the quantity introduced. Nor must we forget the great differences in the ages and in the conditions of health of the patients. The plastic mass poured out from the ciliary body and iris had in many cases enveloped the remains of the lenses (Pl. V., Fig. 31; also Pl. III., Fig. 19), which can be seen in process of disintegration under the action of phago-

PLATE V

FIG. 28: SPECIMEN NO. 130.—The iris shows a deep jagged tear. There are two scars made at the operation, one over the posterior part of the ciliary body, the other near the equator of the eye. Numerous white dots are seen on the choroid and iris.

FIG. 29: SPECIMEN NO. 148.—There is a localised patch of inflammation within the globe behind the equator; in this was found a foreign body, probably the tip of the copper probe used in the operation. It lay in the vitreous cavity within the retina, which is totally detached.

FIG. 30: SPECIMEN NO. 72.—The operation scar can be seen on the temporal side of the sclera behind the equator. The choroid and retina are extensively detached on this side, having evidently been pushed before the instrument before it succeeded in penetrating them. To the nasal side in the anterior part of the vitreous chamber lies a cone of exudate, the apex of which (posteriorly) is adherent to the retina, and has raised it from its bed in the form of a shallow bleb. The cornea fell in during preparation; it was ulcerated. The anterior chamber was full of pus and blood. What is left of the lens lies buried at the base of the cone of exudate already referred to, being bound thereby to the ciliary body and to the back of the iris.

FIG. 31: SPECIMEN NO. 171.—A whole-section of the eye shown in Fig. 19. For details of description refer to that figure.

FIG. 32: SPECIMEN NO. 171.—Low-power magnification of a portion of the specimen shown in the previous figure. To the right is seen the inflamed and matted iris; beneath this lies a mass of inflammatory exudate in which the curled remains of the lens capsule can be traced. In this mass of exudate the lens nucleus lies imbedded, its margins being surrounded by large phagocytes.

FIG. 33: SPECIMEN NO. 171.—High-power magnification of portion of the previous specimen, showing some of the phagocytes much enlarged. Notice their processes invading the lens substance.

PLATE V.

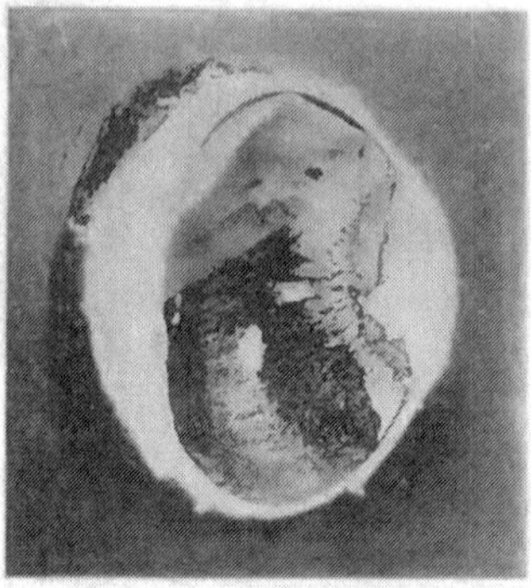

FIG. 28 (No. 130).—Left eye, upper half.

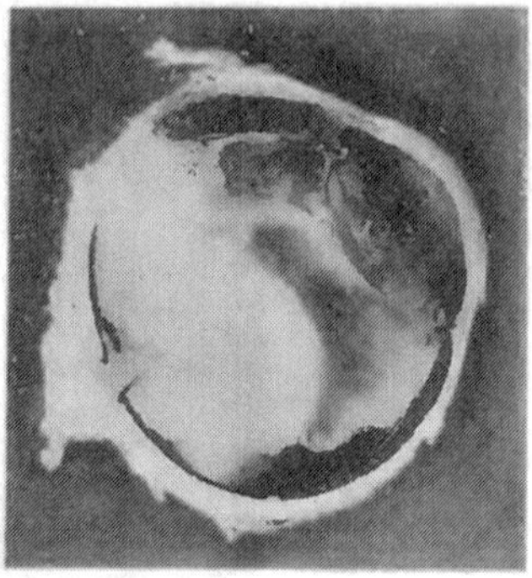

FIG. 29 (No. 148).—Left eye, upper half.

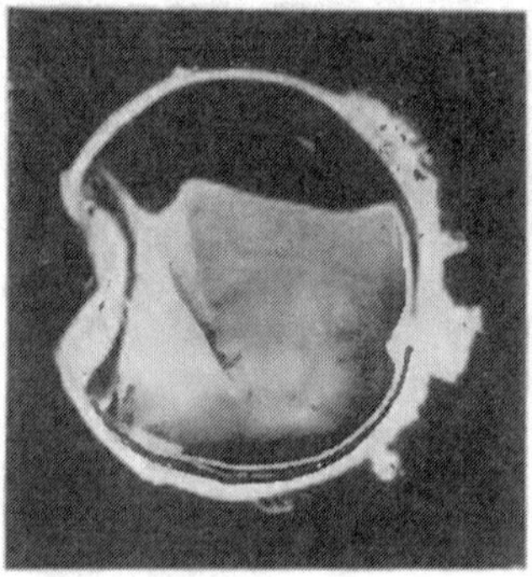

FIG. 30 (No. 72).—Right eye, lower half.

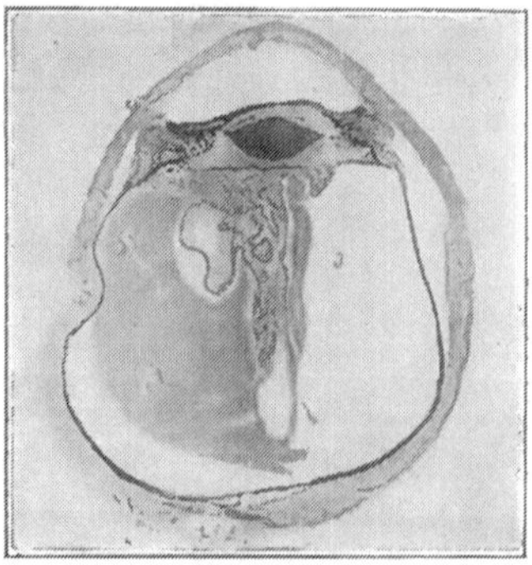

FIG. 31 (No. 171).—Left eye, whole section.

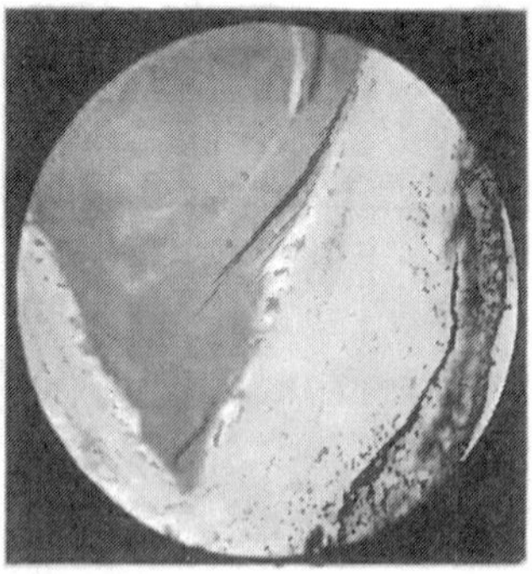

FIG. 32 (No. 171).—Microscopic section, low power.

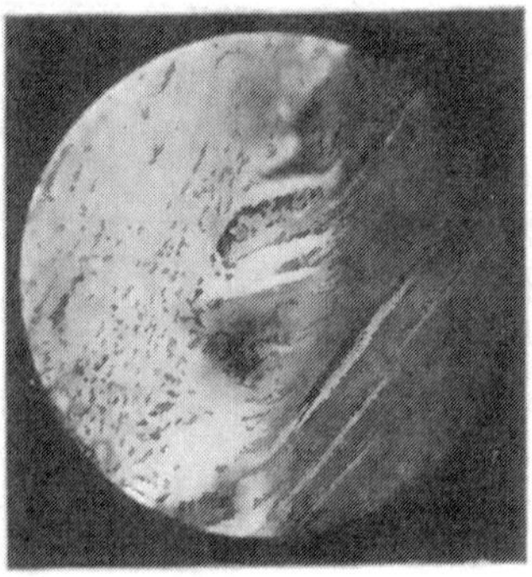

FIG. 33 (No. 171).—Microscopic section, high power.

cytosis (Pl. V., Figs. 32 and 33) or of fluid absorption. Evidence of calcification of the lens was obtained in at least one specimen (Pl. VI., Fig. 35), and the same process was also found at work in the uveal coat of several others. The rupture of the lens capsule often provides a ready path of ingress for the inflammatory exudate, which can then be seen filling the cavity of the capsule as well as surrounding it. The curly remains, both of the anterior and of the posterior portions of the capsule, can be clearly traced in many of the specimens, imbedded in dense masses of organising inflammatory exudate. In several such, the absence of the capsule opposite or to one side of the pupillary area, and the curled-up ends of the elastic membrane, mark the spot where rupture was effected at the time of operation.

In only one instance has any evidence of proliferative uveitis come to light, and in this one the nodule in the iris consists of mononuclear lymphocytes; epithelioid and giant cells are conspicuous by their absence. The interest of this observation centres in the fact that a large number of these globes were removed with the object of guarding against the occurrence of sympathetic ophthalmia, or of making safer the performance of an extraction in the opposite eye. So far as the first indication is concerned, it would appear that the danger of sympathetic mischief in the second eye after couching is not great. The deduction thus drawn from pathological data is confirmed by the author's clinical experience, for, as far as his observations go, it is extremely rare to see the second eye lost by sympathetic ophthalmia after this operation.

The Chambers of the Eye.

The Anterior Chamber.—This chamber showed departures from the normal in different directions. These will be dealt with under separate headings.

1. *Scantiness of Contents.*—One chamber was quite empty, due to the presence of a corneal fistula (Pl. IV., Fig. 23). In a number of cases the chamber was greatly shallowed, owing to the encroachment of the vitreous body upon it. In these the filtering angle was sealed by adhesion over a wide area. In a few cases *l'iris bombé* was responsible for the shallowing

of the chamber (Pl. VI., Fig. 34). In yet others a severe plastic inflammation had involved the structures, lying in and posterior to the aqueous chamber, and had matted them to the posterior surface of the cornea, thus almost obliterating the cavity. This union had been so strong that in the process of hardening the membrane of Descemet remained adherent to the organised exudate beneath it, and a spurious chamber was thus formed lying in the substance of the cornea (Pl. VI., Figs. 35 and 36).

2. *Hypopyon* was present in 6 specimens, and in one the pus was mixed with blood. The length of histories in these cases varied from a matter of months up to twenty years.

3. *Hyphæma.*—Blood was present in the anterior chamber in 9 specimens. In some of them it was fresh, whilst in others it was altered and decolorised. The long histories given by a number of these cases suggest either that there had been some recent cause for hæmorrhage, or else that a leakage of blood had been constantly occurring. In 2 of the eyes the iris had been torn; in every one of the others there was evidence that severe iritis had been present.

4. *Vitreous in the Anterior Chamber.* — In 4 eyeballs the aqueous and vitreous cavities appear to have been in free communication with each other, and filaments of the vitreous body can be traced into the anterior chamber. In 2 of these the angle was widely open, and in the other 2 it was closed by irido-corneal adhesions.

5. *Lens Matter in the Chamber* (Pl. II., *Figs.* 10, 12, *and* 13). —In 4 eyes lens matter was found in the anterior chamber. In one the history showed that a nucleus had passed freely backwards and forwards between the two chambers (Pl. II., Fig. 11). In another a Morgagnian cataract was wedged in the angle of the chamber, but had contracted no adhesions; in the remaining 2 the nuclear masses were firmly fixed in position by an abundant quantity of exudate.

6. *Albuminous Exudates in the Anterior Chamber.*—These were found in 3 cases; few or no structural elements were present. During life the contents of the chamber were fluid, but they had coagulated under the influence of the formalin preparation of the specimens; they were probably derived from the iris and ciliary body.

The Vitreous Chamber.—In the great majority of the

PLATE VI

FIG. 34: SPECIMEN NO. 111.—The anterior chamber is much shallowed by the bulging forward of the iris (l'iris bombé); the pupil is blocked, and its edges are adherent to a layer composed of the lens capsule and the anterior layer of the hyaloid, which are inflamed and matted together. The retina is totally detached, and the choroid partly so. A large cyst can be seen in what was the central region of the retina. It is cut across in the section. (See also Fig. 44.)

FIG. 35: SPECIMEN NO. 74.—From before backward we see (1) the cornea; (2) a space which might be mistaken for the anterior chamber, but which is really an artificial tear in the substance of the cornea (see Fig. 36); (3) the remains of the iris and ciliary body matted in a mass of exudate in which is imbedded (4) what is left of the lens. Large areas of this structure have undergone calcification; the wavy capsule can be seen surrounding the lens remnants. Behind this and continuous with it is a further mass of exudate, which tightly mats the folds of the detached retina to the structures already mentioned.

FIG. 36: SPECIMEN NO. 74.—A higher magnification of a portion of the preceding section. From above downward in the figure we see (1) the cornea; (2) the artificial space; (3) the papillary margins of the iris imbedded in dense exudate. Lining the lower boundary of the space is seen the greatly convoluted membrane of Descemet, which has been torn away from its corneal attachments, having clung more tightly to the exudate, in which the iris is imbedded, than to its normal attachments.

FIG. 37: SPECIMEN NO. 250.—A large Morgagnian cataract lies imbedded in a fine inflammatory exudate into the vitreous cavity; in this exudate are many white inflammatory foci. The retina also shows many white dots, the sclera is staphylomatous, and the anterior chamber is extremely shallow.

FIG. 38: SPECIMEN NO. 72.—The inflamed optic nerve head shows a mass of exudate occupying the physiological cup and bulging into the vitreous cavity. This mass is undergoing organisation, and new-formed vessels are to be seen in it at numerous points; it was the apical end of a conical mass which represented the infiltrated and shrunken vitreous body. Notice the pull of the roots of the mass on the edges of the physiological cup.

FIG. 39.: SPECIMEN NO. 199.—The conical mass occupying the vitreous cavity has here undergone a high degree of organisation, especially towards its apex at the optic nerve and in the neighbourhood of the ora serrata. The canal of Stilling is probably indicated by the white irregular lines seen in the centre of the cone. The pupil is blocked with dense exudate which fuses with that of the cone; the contraction of the latter has completely detached the retina from its bed.

PLATE VI.

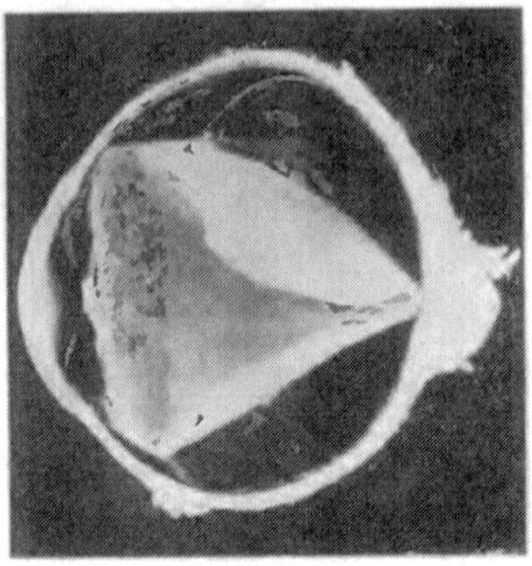

FIG. 34 (No. 111).—Left eye, upper half.

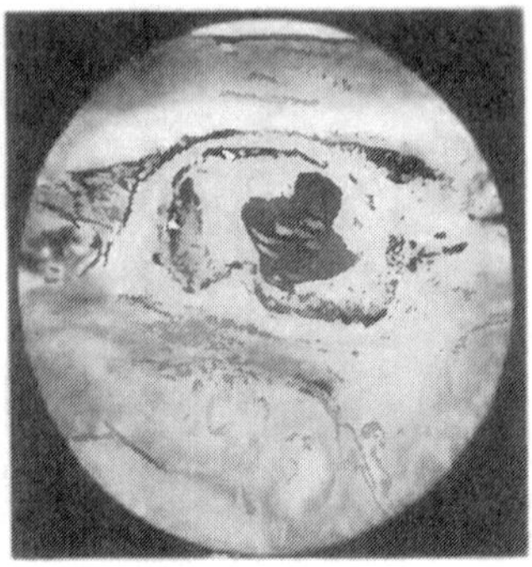

FIG. 35 (No. 74).—Microscopic section, low power.

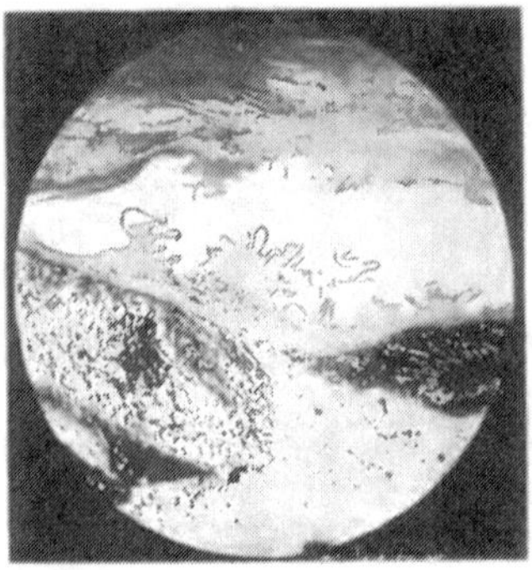

FIG. 36 (No. 74).—Microscopic section, higher power.

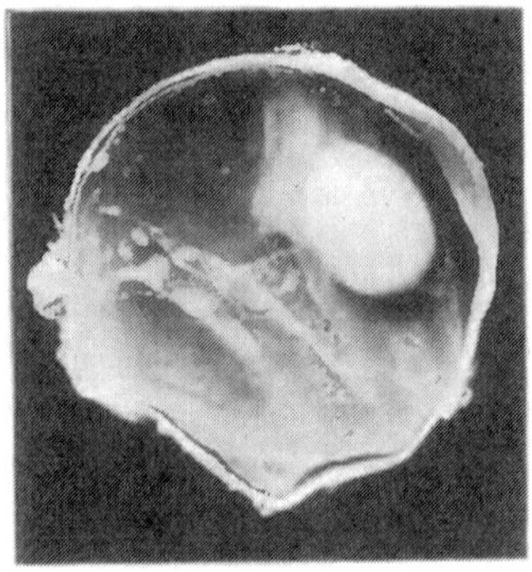

FIG. 37 (No. 250).—Right eye, lower half.

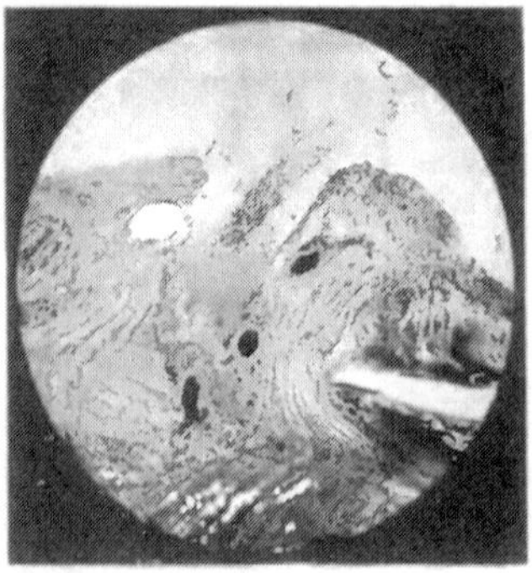

FIG. 38 (No. 72).—Microscopic section, low power.

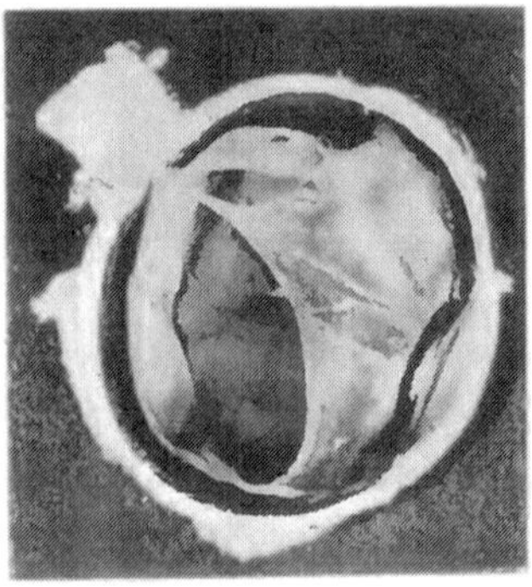

FIG. 39 (No. 199).—Right eye, lower half.

eyeballs under examination, it was observed that the vitreous body had become detached and shrunken, and that its remnants showed distinct signs of infiltration, and often of organisation. The appearances observed in the various cases fall naturally under a number of headings: (1) Very slight evidence of vitreous structure is discernible (Pl. II., Fig. 14). (2) Filmy masses are present in the chamber (Pl. II., Fig. 15). These either (*a*) are confined to the anterior portion of the chamber, or (*b*) take the form of a cone with its apex at the nerve head, and its base in the neighbourhood of the ora serrata and ciliary body. (3) Masses are present which give the impression of being freely infiltrated with inflammatory material, either throughout their substance (Pl. III., Fig. 16) or in isolated foci (Pl. VI., Fig. 37); these may be divided into the same subgroups, (*a*) and (*b*), as those under the previous heading. (4) A distinct fibrous organisation is noticeable in the conical masses, which represent the detached and shrunken vitreous (Pl. III., Fig. 17). (5) No detail is discernible (Pl. III., Fig. 19), owing to the fact that the retina has become detached and inextricably matted with the one-time vitreous contents, and with the iris and ciliary body.

There are certain preliminary points which we must first settle:

1. There is no essential difference between the cases in which there is a definite cone of filmy or infiltrated membrane reaching from the optic nerve head to the ciliary body, and those in which deposits of a similar nature are found confined to the anterior portion of the vitreous chamber. The grounds for this statement are as follows: (*a*) An examination of the more complete specimens of conical exudate shows that the membrane becomes very slender as the nerve head is approached, and it is obvious that very little violence would be required to break this delicate thread across, and so to allow the whole membrane to be gathered up by its own elasticity towards its large and strong anterior attachments. (*b*) There is strong evidence in a number of the specimens of this series to show that the contraction of the shrinking inflammatory material within the globes takes place with such force as might easily suffice to break across the slender nerve attachment of some of these cones. (*c*) It is obvious that in not a few cases the

tapering apex of a conical exudate is likely to be cut across during section of the globe, or broken across during subsequent manipulations. (*d*) Specimens in which the exudates presented a definite conical shape, when they were first cut in India, have arrived in this country transformed during the voyage into the similitude of those in which the exudate is loosely gathered into the fore part of the vitreous chamber; the apex of the cone had been broken off at the nerve head, and the exudate had moved forward by virtue of its own elasticity toward the anterior attachments of the mass. Taking all these points into consideration, we may conclude that in all the eyeballs which present the appearance of shrunken vitreous the structure was originally conical in form, and that departures from that shape are merely artefacts. Stress is laid on this point, because in a number of the globes the appearances present suggest that the exudate is poured out from the ciliary body, and is confined to the neighbourhood of that structure. We believe such an interpretation to be quite erroneous, and to be founded on the observation of artefacts.

2. Is this appearance of a shrunken vitreous body definitely pathological? The answer is in the affirmative, for the following reasons: (*a*) All these globes were treated alike, being dropped into 5 per cent. formalin solution on removal, and kept there till frozen and cut. (*b*) Normal eyeballs treated in this way present no such evidence of definite vitreous structure. (*c*) Every grade can be traced in the series before us, between the appearance of delicate filmy membranes in the vitreous and the presence of firmly organised structures. (*d*) Though it is very difficult to examine these exudates satisfactorily under the microscope, there are a large number of specimens which definitely show evidence of an inflammatory exudation, strengthening and thickening the vitreous body. In not a few of these the anterior hyaloid membrane (the term is used in a non-committal sense) is definitely thickened and infiltrated with inflammatory material (Pl. III., Fig. 20). The conclusion arrived at is that these widely varying evidences of structural alteration in the vitreous body are to be interpreted as due to the penetration of the hyaloid by inflammatory material of chemotaxic

origin, and to the subsequent organisation of that infiltration. (*e*) There still remains the clinical evidence. The author was increasingly reluctant, as his Indian experience accumulated, to remove lenses which had been couched. It was not that vitreous escaped, but that the results of operation were usually poor, and that the blame of the lost sight was then apt to be most unfairly ascribed to the extraction operation. In view of the frequent occurrence of vitreous changes, this failure to help the patients is easily explained. Major Kirkpatrick has taken a different, and possibly a more generous, view of the position, and has removed a number of these couched lenses. His evidence is of extreme interest in the light of our recent pathological findings; he has been " struck by the rarity of vitreous escape even after a fairly extensive investigation with a spoon " in extracting couched lenses. He adds:

" I have noticed that the vitreous body becomes shrunken and extraordinarily tough, so much so that when an eye is excised (either for glaucoma or for iridocyclitis following Mahomedan operation), the whole globe can be held up by a strabismus hook transfixing the vitreous, though the latter appears perfectly clear. The vitreous undoubtedly does undergo shrinkage, and leaves a large space, which is occupied by aqueous."

Straub* has described some experiments which he made on animals, in the course of which he injected pathogenic organisms either into the vitreous or into the ciliary body. The result varied according to the part infected, and the poisoned area attracted leucocytes by chemotaxis to itself. Particular interest attaches to the following of his findings: (1) The optic nerve head was swollen and filled up with leucocytes; (2) there was evidence " that the lymph current of the vitreous goes by the optic nerve, and that chemotaxic substances are brought by this current from the granuloma (the artificial infection) to the nerve "; (3) the leucocytes found in the vitreous showed the way from the granuloma to the cup of the optic nerve—they were seated on thin membranes, and most of them were heaped together in small dots; (4) aggregations were found

* "The Pathology of Dust-like Bodies in the Vitreous," etc., Trans. of the O.S. of the U.K., 1912, xxxii. 60.

on the walls of the cavities of the eye (on the cornea, on the retina, on the lens capsule, etc.), attracted there, in Straub's opinion, by a chemotaxic action.

In the experiments above considered, which were very limited in number, an effort was made to localise the infection to one or other part of the eye, and to work with a virus (tubercle bacilli) which was comparatively constant in its toxicity.

What Straub did with a few eyes has been done in the series now before us, by the Indian coucher, in fifty-four. The interest of the experiments is heightened by the fact that, whereas in the Dutch experiments the toxicity of the virus was kept as constant as possible, in the Indian ones it varied from that of organisms which took many years to destroy the sight to that of one which at once produced a fulminating panophthalmitis. One point more: The Indian operator made no effort to confine his procedure (and with that procedure went infection) to any one structure; sometimes he attacked the lens from in front, and in doing so he often primarily injured the iris, but may have spared the vitreous chamber; sometimes he entered through the ciliary body or through the choroid, opening up the hyaloid cavity in doing so. His want of skill and the slenderness of his anatomical knowledge made him catholic in the damage he inflicted, but running through his work is the trail of septic infection of the eyeball by penetrating wounds. The result is that he has provided us with a large material of extraordinary interest in the study of the problem which Straub started on.

The Filmy Masses in the Vitreous Chamber.—As has already been stated, the contents of the vitreous chamber in these specimens vary from thin gauzy films, which can only be detected by careful search, up to thick masses which strike the eye as soon as the specimen is looked at.

It is not easy to obtain a view of these exudates in section, but nevertheless they appear in a considerable number of the microscopic specimens, and their character is always the same; they consist of more or less structureless masses with blood-cells and leucocytes imbedded in their substance. In fact, they would seem to be identical with the membrane spoken of by Straub as harbouring the leucocytes which gave rise to dust-like and other opacities of the vitreous in his experimental cases. At a later stage, or perhaps in cases where the inflammation has been of a more plastic character, a distinct fibrillation of the exudate can be seen, and there may even be evidence of a definite fibrous tissue formation. If we confine our attention for the moment to those eyeballs in which the exuded mass is devoid of structure in the anterior portion of the cone, we shall find that, on tracing it back toward the apex by which it is attached to the optic nerve, it becomes more highly organised and more richly cellular, whilst fibrillation and fibrous tissue formation make their appearance. The same thing, though in a lesser degree, may be observed in the neighbourhood of the ciliary body, doubtless due to the presence of a plastic exudate derived from that structure.

An examination (Pl. VI., Fig. 38) of the optic nerve and of the exudate attached to it reveals the following features: (1) The nerve head is congested, and its vessels stand out in prominent relief. (2) There is a considerable effusion of leucocytes in the neighbourhood of these vessels. (3) A mass of exudate fills up and projects from the optic nerve cup, whether this latter is physiological or glaucomatous. This mass is clearly contracting, and thereby pulling on the tissue which lines the edges of the cup. (4) Along the centre of the projecting exudate are to be seen (*a*) an abundance of mononuclear cells; (*b*) the commencement of a fibrous tissue formation; and (*c*) a new formation of bloodvessels.

The appearances above enumerated would indicate that we have to do with an inflammation of the optic nerve, which had been induced by chemotaxic substances brought thither along Stilling's canal. Such an idea is not a new one. It was suggested by Straub in order to explain the optic neuritis he found in his two cases of experimental inoculations of the ciliary body, and it also enjoys provisionally the support of Fuchs's* authority. The idea that part of the lymph of the eye passes backward along a passage corresponding to the central hyaloid canal is not generally accepted, and rests largely on inference from the observation of pathological specimens. It would be difficult, however, for anyone who

* Fuchs: "Textbook of Ophthalmology" Duane, fourth edition. 1911, p. 16.

has carefully studied this series to doubt that such a flow exists; it is, of course, not suggested that any large percentage of the lymph travels in this direction.

A confirmation of these views is obtained if we refer to the three eyeballs in which the organisation of the cone of exudate into the vitreous has attained the highest development. We notice in these how extremely far this process of organisation has been carried in the apex of the cone, where it is represented as a well-defined opaque cord (Pl. VI., Fig. 39; and Pl. III., Fig. 17). In one of the three a fibrous band, presumably the remains of the canal of Stilling, is clearly seen, whilst in the two others the existence of this structure is at least indicated. It is possible that in the first-named a congenital peculiarity exaggerated the distinctness of the appearance.

The Retina.

Detachment of the retina occurred in 38 of the 54 globes (70·38 per cent.), and was absent in 16 (29·62 per cent.). It was partial and ill-marked in 5 (9·25 per cent.), extensive in 9 (16·68 per cent.), and complete in 24 (44·44 per cent.). The ocular tension was above normal in 11 out of the 16, which presented no detachment, but in only 6 out of the remaining 38; it was below the normal in 13 of the 24 globes with complete detachment, and above it in 3 of them. In the very great majority of the eyes the detachment of the retina was undoubtedly due to traction from within. The sequence of events is plain from a study of the whole series.

At the operation there was an infection of the coats of the eye, and also of the vitreous chamber from without; this led to the formation of inflammatory material within the vitreous chamber; adhesions took place between these new-formed membranes and the retina; finally the shrinkage of the organising inflammatory material tore the retina from its bed. Every step of the process can be traced either in microscopic sections or in the naked-eye specimens. The earliest possible stage is seen under the microscope in sections of an eyeball (No. 37), where in the neighbourhood of the ora serrata the shrinkage of the exudate within the vitreous chamber has just begun to lift the retina from its bed. The individual points of attachment between the inflammatory membrane and the retina are beautifully illustrated. The ultimate stage of the process is to be found in those cases in which the retina is not merely totally detached, but has shrunk posteriorly into a stick-like form (Pl. III., Fig. 19, and Pl. IV., Fig. 25), whilst it opens out anteriorly into a mass in which the iris, the ciliary body, the lens, the remains of the vitreous, and the retina are inextricably matted and tangled. When sections of such specimens are examined under the microscope, their leading feature is the evidence of severe plastic iridocyclitis, with the formation of abundant cicatricial tissue, which mats all the parts together and severely distorts the normal anatomical arrangement. The retina is dragged forward from the neighbourhood of the ora serrata over the ciliary body, whilst elsewhere it is thrown into abundant folds and completely separated from its normal attachments. A pseudo-cystic condition is thus produced, the apparent cysts being formed by the elaborate folding of the membrane (Pl. III., Fig. 19, and Pl. V., Fig. 31). These may be small and slit-like, or may be large and round, so simulating the appearance of true cysts. In front of the retinal mass, lens fragments and capsule are seen in a number of the specimens entangled in the scar-tissue. As has already been said, all grades can be traced, from the slightest detachments up to those we have just been describing. The greater or less degree of separation of the retina met with in the different globes is doubtless in part a question of time, but it is also, and probably to a much larger extent, one of the character and grade of the inflammatory process excited in the eyeball. The more plastic the type of inflammation and the more intense the process is, the greater will be the measure of ultimate cicatrisation, always provided that the inflammation is not intense enough to result in suppuration.

There are several different ways in which the exudate which forms within the vitreous chamber may be placed in a favourable position for the production of retinal detachment.

1. The first of these is illustrated by each of those globes (Nos. 44 and 72) in which the site of a wound of the retina forms the point of connection between that membrane and

the inflammatory exudate lying in the vitreous cavity (Pl. V., Fig. 30). The traumatic infection of the retina served to attach the vitreous exudate to its walls, and thus paved the way for the separation of the membrane. In one of these cases (No. 44) a longitudinal fold was detached, whilst in the other (No. 72) the detachment was broad and shallow.

2. In the second method also, it is necessary to postulate an infection of the retina before that membrane could have contracted adhesions, either localised or widespread, to the neighbouring vitreous exudate. Once, however, the virus was planted within the hyaloid chamber, it probably diffused itself widely, and by means of chemotaxis set up an inflammation of the retina; evidences of such a retinitis abound in many of the specimens. Attachments between the vitreous exudate and the retina having been thus formed, the contraction of the former would naturally lead to the separation of the latter from its choroidal bed.

3. In a few of the globes the contracting membrane is merely an infiltration and thickening of the anterior layer of the hyaloid. It is well known that the vitreous body is, under normal conditions, more firmly attached to the retina in the neighbourhood of the ora serrata than it is elsewhere; it is therefore obvious that an inflammatory contracting membrane in the anterior part of the vitreous will pull throughout its whole circumference on the retina in its neighbourhood, effecting a detachment over a very wide area (Pl. III., Fig. 20). This is just what we see happening in the globes we are now discussing.

4. In a number of the specimens it can be clearly seen that the bands, which drag upon the retina, radiate from the remains of lens masses, which are themselves encased in inflammatory tissue, and are bound thereby to the iris and ciliary body in their neighbourhood. Such bands appear in some cases to lie in the substance of the retina itself (Pl. IV., Fig. 24); in others they are situate in the vitreous and present the form of membranous sheets, separated from the subjacent retina only by narrow spaces, and finding attachment to it in the neighbourhood of the equator (Nos. 117 and 170). The characteristic of these cases would appear to be that the dislocated lens is in them the principal focus of sepsis within the

eye. The point is of interest, since some of them, at least, represent ruptured Morgagnian cataracts; for there is reason to believe, on clinical grounds, that the liberation of Morgagnian fluid within the eye is, sometimes at least, productive of considerable irritation to the surrounding parts.

There are two globes in the collection in which the exudate within the hyaloid cavity, converted into organised fibrous tissue, is obviously tearing the retina from its bed in the course of its contraction. A very interesting feature of these eyeballs is that in each of them an opaque band which strongly suggests Stilling's canal can be traced forward from the optic nerve head (Pl. VI., Fig. 39).

In many of the specimens an abundant subretinal exudate is present. In the long-standing ones, with complete detachment of the retina, this effusion fills up the whole of the space between the retina and the choroid. When the latter membrane is also detached, a further exudate of similar appearance is seen between it and the sclera. Owing to the action of the formalin, the very firm coagulation of the long-standing effusions gives the eyes a solid and very characteristic appearance (Pl. III., Fig. 19); the half-globes look like sections of marbles made of fissured and clouded glass. In earlier cases the effused mass is much less firm, but is whiter and more opaque, with a tendency to present a flocculent appearance. The question that naturally presents itself is, whether these effusions were the cause or the result of the retinal detachment. The presence of the inflammatory exudate within the vitreous, with which we have already dealt, provides such a satisfactory explanation of the detachments of the retina throughout this series, that it seems unlikely that the effusions in question, whether subretinal or subchoroidal, play any causative part whatever.

We must place in quite a different category the cases, four in number, in which the effused fluid consisted of blood. The source of the hæmorrhage in these cases is different from that which is met with when the pressure within an eye is suddenly reduced by the operative opening of the globe. In the latter case it is the large choroidal vessels which give way, and the hæmorrhage is subchoroidal, whereas in the four cases under review the bleeding was subretinal in one (No. 157), into the vitreous chamber alone in one (Pl. VII., Fig. 40), and into both the vitreous chamber and the subretinal space in two. The hæmorrhage into the vitreous chamber was probably due to injury to the retinal vessels by the coucher's instrument, though it is possible that blood may have found its way through the retinal cut from choroidal vessels divided at the time. The subretinal hæmorrhage probably escaped from the severed branches of the smaller choroidal vessels. The fact that in no case was a large subchoroidal hæmorrhage present would indicate that the large choroidal vessels were tough enough to escape injury, being probably pushed aside by the comparatively blunt instrument the coucher used. In one eyeball (No. 157) large cholesterine crystals were seen shining on the cut surface of the sanguineous mass. A similar phenomenon was observed in the case of one of the albuminous effusions above spoken of.

It remains to deal with a rare cause of detachment of the retina or of the retina and choroid—viz., the application of direct violence at the time of operation. This is best exemplified in the two globes in which the cataract was thrust through and behind the retina, by the coucher's instrument, at the time of operation (Pl. IV., Fig. 22). It is also beautifully illustrated by specimen No. 72, in which the retina and choroid were carried in front of the coucher's instrument before the latter succeeded in perforating them (Pl. V., Fig. 30). The dislocation thus produced proved permanent.

Dots on the Retina.—A striking feature of the series of specimens before us is the presence of numerous dots on the retina. These are to be seen in 16 cases, and doubtfully in a seventeenth. In at least one other, similar dots are present on the choroid and on the posterior surface of the iris (Pl. V., Fig. 28). We therefore find this peculiar appearance in one case in every three; but this is far from representing what is probably its real relative frequency, for in 24 of the globes the retina was totally detached, and it was therefore impossible to say whether there were dots present on it or not. If we put these 24 to one side, we find that the dots were certainly present in 16 out of 30—that is, in well over 50 per cent. If we include the other 2 cases above alluded to, the figure rises to 60 per cent.

In some of the specimens the dots are so large that they could scarcely be missed under a careful naked-eye examination (Pl. III., Fig. 18), whilst in others they were only discovered when highly magnified photographs of the eyeballs were thrown on a screen (Pl. III., Fig. 17). They could, however, be found easily with a loupe once their presence was known. The variation in different specimens was not confined to size; some of the dots were white, others were a pale grey, and a few were bright and shiny. Again, some of them appeared much more sharply defined than others.

It was at first thought that manifestations so distinct under slight magnification would yield very definite appearances under the microscope; but, on the contrary, much difficulty has been experienced in deciding the nature of the changes which have given rise to this phenomenon.

One of the first points noticed was that the dots were found almost exclusively in long-standing cases. This of itself would appear to indicate that their cause was to be sought in some degenerative process; but a closer analysis of the histories revealed a probable fallacy in such an argument, since a number of the eyes had had good vision for a long period after operation, and had eventually succumbed to a fresh inflammatory invasion, or possibly to a more severe recrudescence of a septic condition implanted at the time of operation.

On examination of a number of specimens, three distinct appearances have been found, any one of which might presumably account for the dots seen with the naked eye.

1. In some of the globes a proliferative retinitis can be found along certain of the vessels (Pl. VII., Fig. 41). These consist in section of masses of mononuclear leucocytes surrounding the vessel wall, and tending to make their way to the inner surface of the retina. It might be thought that such a change would produce lines rather than dots, and that those lines would run along the course of the vessels; but there are two features which make this doubtful: (*a*) Even under the same field some of the vessels appear quite healthy on section, whilst others show distinct masses of proliferation; and (*b*) along

the course of a vessel cut obliquely one may find the proliferative exudate confined to one part of its course, the rest being comparatively free.

2. In the neighbourhood of some of the inflamed retinal vessels above spoken of, one finds on the surface of the retina what appear to be free collections of mononuclear cells (Pl. VII., Fig. 42). These are apparently of the same nature as the dots described by Straub on the posterior surface of the cornea and in the vitreous body. It will be remembered that he attributed them to chemotaxic action. It would appear not improbable that the same explanation holds for these retinal dots. It is of interest that, though they occur in cases of long standing, the history of a subsequent inflammation, destructive to vision is of a much later, and indeed, of a comparatively recen date. The presence of such exudative masses would then be easily explained.

3. The grouping of these dots varies considerably in different specimens, but does not lend much colour to the idea that they are vascular in origin, for in some at least of the eyes they certainly do not follow the course of the vessels. On the other hand, in a few of the eyeballs there is a massing of these dots in the neighbourhood of the ora serrata, which is in itself suggestive of a degenerative process, since this is the area of lowest circulatory activity, inasmuch as this region is supplied by the ultimate twigs of the retinal vessels. This observation gathers interest from the fact that in quite a number of these specimens it is possible to demonstrate the presence of small cysts in the walls of the retina (Pl. VII., Fig. 43). These cysts are produced by the coalescence of œdematous spaces in degenerative areas. All stages of the process can be traced in different specimens of the series before us. Such cysts are only likely to be met with in long-standing cases in which the degenerative processes have had time for full play.

Inasmuch as these retinal dots are found in the cases in which the retina is still in its normal position, it would seem probable that a careful clinical search should reveal their presence in living eyes now that their existence is established pathologically. It is a point which should repay the study of surgeons who are practising where couching is commonly resorted to, and especially in India.

PLATE VII

FIG. 40: SPECIMEN NO. 240.—The original cavity of the vitreous is represented by a mass of blood-clot, surrounded by the walls of the totally detached retina. The subretinal exudate is firm and abundant. The iris and ciliary body, the lens remnants, and the anterior part of the retina are matted together in a dense mass of cicatricial tissue.

FIG. 41: SPECIMEN NO. 175.—This shows a proliferative dot in the retina. R, retina; SCL, sclera; CH, choroid; D, mass of leucocytes surrounding vessel wall.

FIG. 42: SPECIMEN NO. 37.—A collection of leucocytes lying on the inner surface of the retina, superficial to its limiting membrane, and projecting freely into the vitreous. In the substance of the retina can be seen the section of a vessel surrounded by a mass of leucocytes.

FIG. 43: SPECIMEN NO. 111.—Small cysts in the retina, which would probably have coalesced before long to form a larger one.

FIG. 44: SPECIMEN NO. 111.—A whole-section of the eye already shown in Fig. 34. The condition of l'iris bombé is well marked, the pupillary edges being adherent to an inflammatory mass formed of the capsule and the anterior layers of the hyaloid matted together. Notice the large cysts occupying the central area of the detached retina, with the macula lutea showing in its inner wall.

FIG. 45: SPECIMEN NO. 131.—A large Morgagnian lens in its capsule was adherent to the iris base, the ciliary body, and the neighbouring retina over a wide area. The capsule ruptured during the transit of the specimen from India. Note the thickened white dots upon it; they are characteristic of Morgagnian cataract. The large brown nucleus, which escaped when the capsule burst, now lies free in the cavity of the eye; notice the "bite" out of its edge. The optic disc was deeply cupped, and the angle of the anterior chamber was widely obliterated, the chamber itself being very shallow.

PLATE VII.

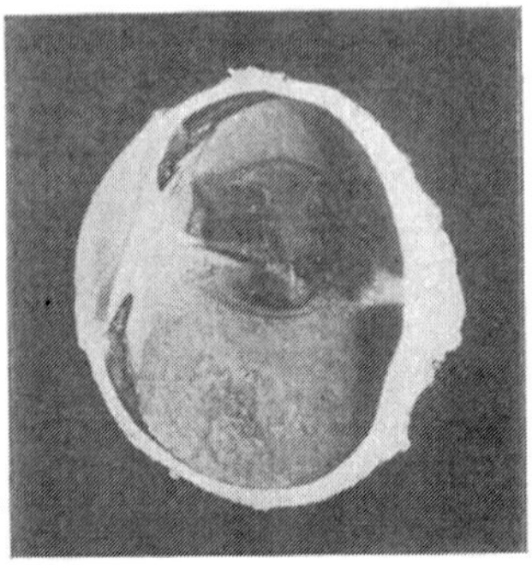

FIG. 40 (No. 240).—Left eye, lower half.

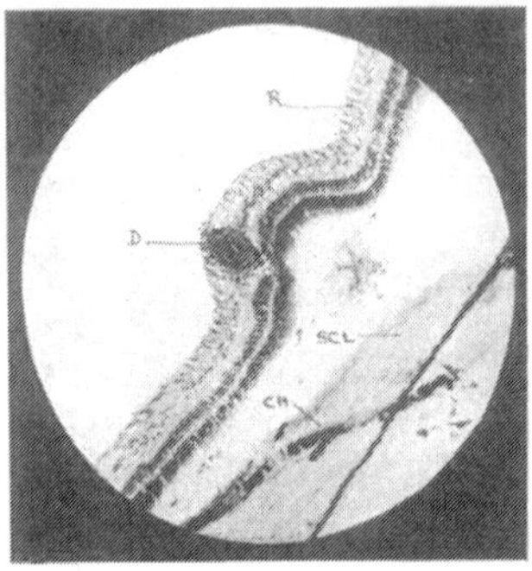

FIG. 41 (No. 175).—Microscopic section, low power.

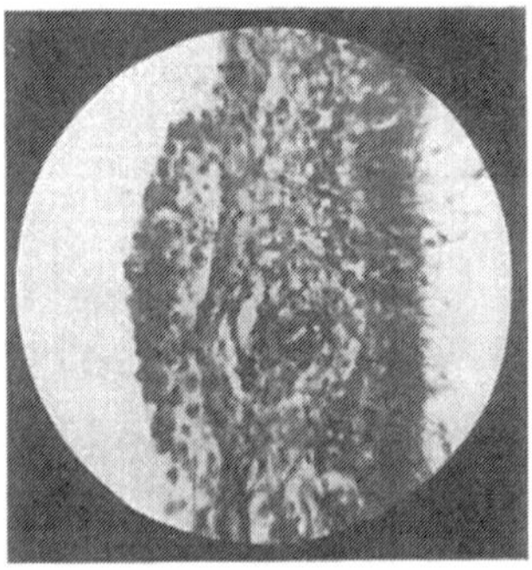

FIG. 42 (No. 37).—Microscopic section, high power.

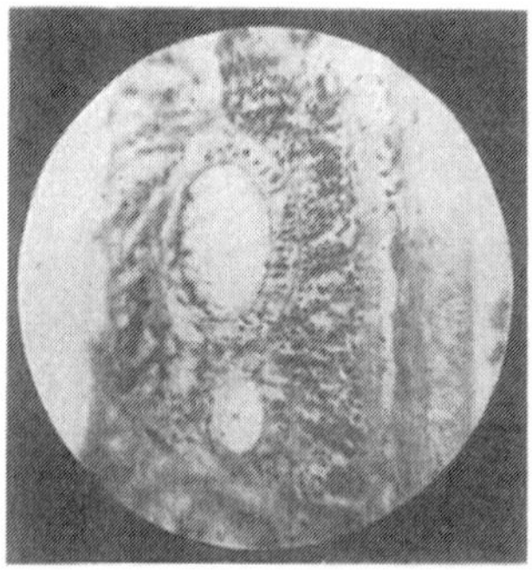

FIG. 43 (No. 111).—Cysts in retina. Microscopic section, high power.

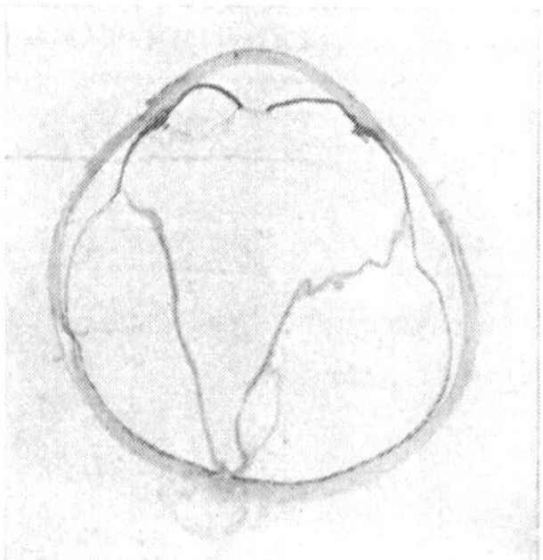

FIG. 44 (No. 111).—Left eye, whole section.

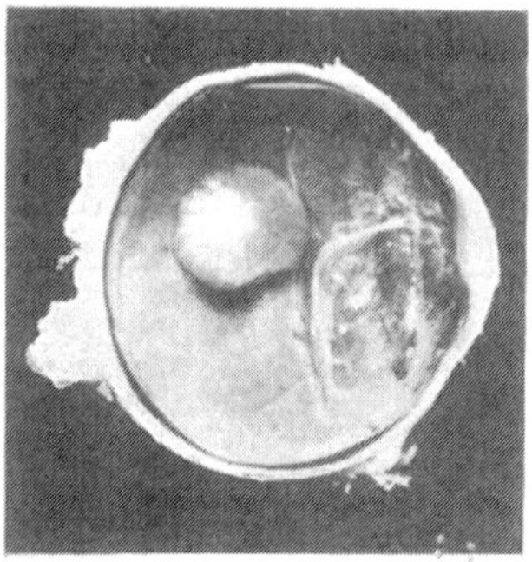

FIG. 45 (No. 131).—Left eye, lower half.

Macroscopic Cysts of the Retina.—It remains to speak of larger cysts of the retina which can be recognised by the naked eye. It has already been mentioned that, in those cases in which this membrane has been found to be tightly folded on itself, a pseudo-cystic condition is thereby produced; the cavities of these false cysts are merely shut-off portions of the original vitreous chamber. Of a quite different nature are the true cysts of the retina, three examples of which are to be found in this collection. In one (Pl. II., Fig. 12) a narrow slit-like cyst is seen in the outer layers of the detached retina at its lower part. In the second, a whole-section of the globe shows a large cyst occupying the central region, the macular area forming a portion of its wall (Pl. VII., Fig. 44). Lastly, in the third a large round cyst can be seen to the temporal side. A point of interest in connection with this specimen is that it shows both true and false retinal cysts (Pl. III., Fig. 19, and Pl. V., Fig. 31).

The Choroid.

It remains to add a few words to what has already been said about this membrane. The great majority of the changes we have found in it are, clearly, to be attributed to the effects either of hypertony or of hypotony of the eye; they do not, therefore, differ from similar appearances found under the same conditions generally.

Compared with detachments of the retina, those of the choroid are rare in this series. In one instance, already mentioned, the two membranes had been displaced together by the instrument used in couching (Pl. V., Fig. 30). In another, in which severe inflammation had occurred, the retina and choroid had adhered to each other, and had been detached as one sheet by the contraction of an exudate, which lay in the neighbourhood of the iris and ciliary body and in the front part of the vitreous cavity. In a number of other globes, in which the tension was low, the ciliary body and the anterior portion of the choroid were found separated from the sclera as far back as the line where the anterior segment of the latter coat was drawn over the posterior in the manner pointed out by Treacher Collins in his work on Hypotony (Trans. of the O.S. of the U.K., 1917).

In the previous chapter we have spoken of an appearance commonly seen in successfully couched eyes—viz., an unusual distinctness of the large vessels of the choroid in the ophthalmoscopic picture. It is necessary to insist that in such cases the vessels are not sclerosed; they are seen with unusual distinctness simply because the pigment which usually hides them from view has disappeared. What is more, a careful study of a number of these cases has created a strong impression that the deficiency in pigmentation affects both the pigmentary layer of the retina and also the pigment of the choroid. The absence of the former lays bare what lies behind it; the absence of the latter is inferred from the general appearance of pseudo-albinism. These findings are the more noteworthy by reason of their contrast to the usual deep pigmentation of the Indian eye. Some of our specimens throw light on this phenomenon, for we observe in them two changes: (1) The pigmentary layer of the retina is irregularly thinned and altered, and at some points its pigment can be seen migrating into the choroid; (2) the choroidal pigment itself is extensively altered in an irregular manner, being heaped up in some areas and thinned in others. It is necessary to remember that, inasmuch as our specimens are wholly obtained from the coucher's failures, whilst the interesting appearance we are discussing is best seen in his successes, we cannot expect very definite results from our pathological material, since the changes we desire to study are there overlaid and obscured by those of pathological processes, such as hypertony, hypotony, and inflammation.

Glaucoma.

It has long been known that couching is frequently followed by secondary glaucoma. In the present series of 54 globes, 19 of them showed evidence of high intra-ocular pressure. This figure must not, however, be taken as a reliable index of the numerical frequency of glaucoma as a complication of the operation. On the one hand, we must remember that the present series deals with the failures only, and that a large number of eyes are met with clinically in which the lens is floating free in the vitreous chamber without any sign that the intra-ocular tension is raised. Again, the cases which go on to suppuration, and which are very numerous, are excluded from the present series owing to the fact that all such were eviscerated in order to avoid the risk of intracranial sepsis. This obviously diminishes the total number of globes under consideration, and thereby raises the apparent percentage of other conditions, such as glaucoma. On the other hand, it would be a mistake to suppose that out of these 54 globes only 19 had suffered from secondary glaucoma, for in 24 of them a complete detachment of the retina had covered up any evidence which may at some time have existed of the presence of increased intra-ocular pressure, though the conditions still found in some of them make it more than probable that the globes were formerly glaucomatous. In any case, it leaves us with the fact that, out of 30 eyeballs which were available for accurate examination, no less than 19 were glaucomatous. In 17 of the 19 the angle of the anterior chamber was extensively closed, and in 3 of these the chamber was so shallow as almost to be reduced to a potential slit. The remaining 2 are thus accounted for: In one the angle was open save for a small marginal adhesion, and there was free communication between the aqueous and vitreous chambers; unfortunately, the specimen was almost spoilt in sectioning it for the microscope; in the second, a Morgagnian lens was impacted in and had blocked the angle of the anterior chamber.

Returning to the 17 cases in which the angle of the chamber was closed, and to certain other eyeballs in which it seemed probable that glaucoma had at some time been present, we found that in every one of them one or other of the accepted causes of secondary glaucoma was revealed when looked for; in some, more than one such cause was discoverable. We shall content ourselves with enumerating these factors.

A corneal fistula, with evidence of past anterior staphyloma, was present in one; here the cause of the glaucoma was evidently the closure of the filtering angle, which resulted from the anterior synechia; in one there was a capsulo-corneal synechia (Pl. IV., Fig. 24), and in another a retino-corneal synechia (Pl. IV., Fig. 25); in 5 the ciliary body was involved in the scar; in 6 the dislocated lens pressed extensively on the iris base (Pl. VII., Fig. 45); in 3 the lenses, tilted at right angles to their normal position, pressed the anterior hyaloid membrane severely back on the side of the dislocation, whilst causing the vitreous to bulge the iris forward into the anterior chamber on the opposite side; in 5 the pupil was blocked, and in 3 of these l'iris bombé was present; in 2 the anterior layers of the hyaloid were so thickened by inflammatory exudate as to suggest that there was an abnormal obstruction to the passage of fluid across the membrane; in one a marked thickening of the lens capsule in the form of an after-cataract may possibly have provided an obstruction to the forward passage of fluid from the vitreous; lastly, there is one globe in which glaucoma had probably been present before the operation, if one may judge from the history of the case and from the violent hæmorrhage which followed the couching.

It has been suggested that one of the causes of glaucoma after this operation is an advance of the front part of the vitreous body owing to a rupture of the anterior layers of the hyaloid during the operation. Without in any way denying that the suggestion may be a valid one in certain cases, the impression gained from a study of this series is that we need look no farther than the well-recognised causes of secondary glaucoma. We have only to remember that the trauma inflicted is extensive and various, and that a greater or less degree of sepsis accompanies every couching in the hands of its Indian exponents.

CHAPTER VI

DIAGNOSIS

THE diagnosis of a case of couched cataract presents the surgeon with three distinct problems: (1) To ascertain whether a couching has been done or not; (2) to discover the new position of the lens and its condition; and (3) to decide whether it is advisable to operate. Only those who work in lands, where the couching of cataracts is an everyday occurrence, will take a deep concern in such questions; but the subject has a scientific interest which cannot fail to appeal to any one who devotes his serious attention to the large questions of ophthalmology.

It might be thought that the simple and obvious way to ascertain whether a couching had been done would be to ask the patient or his relatives. In a large number of cases this is of course sufficient; but in India, at all events, there are many who will deny the operation they have undergone. This is due to the fact that it is widely known among the people that the British surgeons view the coucher and all his methods with extreme disfavour. Patients are therefore reluctant to admit having consulted him, and they also are afraid lest treatment should be refused them, once their true history is known; for it is common knowledge amongst them that the Western practitioner is extremely reluctant to interfere with an eye which a coucher has spoilt. It is well, therefore, to consider carefully the grounds on which the physical diagnosis of a couched lens should rest.

We will first consider the case of those eyes in which **the cataract has been definitely removed from the neighbourhood of the pupil.** These present certain well-marked signs: (1) *The pupil is brilliantly black,* and (2) *the plane of the iris is flat.* It may seem strange to insist upon these points, but to the trained eye they are so obvious that a diagnosis can often be made, as soon as the patient takes his seat in the out-patient room, in front of the surgeon. The quality of the blackness of the pupil is difficult to put into words, but it arrests the attention by its contrast to the ordinary appearance of the pupil in people so advanced in life as the subjects of cataract usually are. The phenomenon is due to the whole cataract, capsule and all, being thrust away from the pupillary area, and it can be equally well seen in cases which have undergone the intra-capsular operation. Then, with regard to the flattening of the iris, the trained eye is used to the appearance presented by the slight forward convexity of that membrane as a result of the presence of the lens behind it; whereas the complete removal, not merely of the lens, but also of the support of the suspensory ligament, makes the iris flatten out in its own plane.

On close inspection we notice other signs. (3) *The iris*, deprived of the support of the lens, *is often tremulous.* This can best be observed if the patient is bidden to move his eye sharply in different directions. (4) *Scars* may be seen *on the iris.* These are the result of tears of the membrane during the operation. In some cases they are associated with an irregularity of the pupil, which may be extreme, or with a limitation or absence of pupillary movements. In other cases the immobility of the pupil, which may be absolute, is associated with (5) *an atrophic condition of the inner free margin of the iris.* Such a condition is only met with in very long-standing cases. Transillumination of the eye will sometimes show up the scars, or the atrophic condition just referred to, as light spaces against the rest of the dark background of the iris. (6) A careful study of the cornea, or of the sclera in its neighbourhood, will often reveal *evidence of the wound made by the instrument* during couching. In the cornea these take the form of small nebulæ or leucomata, lying just within the limbus, and usually in the temporal quadrant. In one case a persistent fistula was met with, as the result, presumably, of the bursting of a staphyloma along the original track of a septic wound. Scars in the sclera are much more difficult to distinguish, but they can sometimes be detected by the pigmentation which overlies them; such pigmentation may be due to the inclusion of uveal pigment in the track of the wound, as has been shown by our pathological specimens: but this is not the only possible explanation of the discoloration, for in dark-skinned races a certain amount of pigmentation is not uncommon after injuries of the conjunctiva. In one of the eyes we examined, there was a filtering scar over a fistula which had formed along the track of a scleral wound. (7) We come now to the leading feature in the diagnosis of these cases—viz., *the recognition of the displaced cataract in its new position* within the eye. In the rare event of a lens being dislocated into the anterior chamber and fixed there, its presence can be easily recognised. Again, in a large number of the cases which present themselves in the out-patient room, the cataract can be seen floating freely in the vitreous, and bobbing up and down with the movements of the eye. In the case of the milky Morgagnian cataracts, or of those cortico-nuclear cataracts which present a glistening and pearly-sectored appearance, it would be difficult even for a beginner to fail to see the lens, which usually lies at the lowest part of the eye. As the patient sits in front of the surgeon, the gleam of the white cataract can be caught each time he looks downward, even though a distance of two or three feet may separate him from the observer. In the case of darker cataracts, such as the pigmented nuclear ones, frequently met with in Indian practice, a closer examination is required.

The patient must be brought nearer to the observer, and facing a good source of illumination. The surgeon then focusses the light on the pupil by the aid of a lens, bidding the patient at the same time to look downward. If this fails, the patient is instructed to bend his head forward, holding the face horizontal; the surgeon then places one closed fist on the back of his head, and gives a number of sharp raps on it with his other fist; when this is done, it is often found that the lens has floated forward on to the pupil. If the patient's head be now quietly raised, the lens can be seen dropping gently away from the pupil, which turns from white or brown (according to the nature of the cataract) to black as it does so. The experiment can be repeated again and again. Sometimes the lens falls away from the pupil so quickly that the surgeon must stoop down and look up at the eye in order to see it. If even after this test he fails to see the cataract, it is safe to assume that it is tied down in its new position by inflammatory adhesions excited by the septic matter introduced at the time of operation. Such adhesions may consist merely of delicate fibrils of exudate, which slightly increase the consistency of the vitreous body, and so to a small extent limit the excursions of the lens; or they may be represented by firm and highly organised fibrous tissue, which mats the lens in its new position, and which may be so strong that even a post-mortem dissection would fail to disengage the cataract from its adventitious position. This subject has been dealt with much more fully in the chapter on pathology. The dilatation of the pupil by a mydriatic will often make it quite easy to discover the whereabouts of the cataract, especially if a strong light, whether natural or artificial, is focussed on the eye by means of a lens. Natural light is preferable to artificial if possible, especially in a country like India, where powerful daylight can be counted on during a large part of the year. The advantage of the white light is especially marked when dealing with brown or dark-coloured cataracts. An examination with the ophthalmoscope or with a transilluminator may sometimes be of value, but in the class of cases we are now discussing, these are seldom of much use, if the examination just described fails to reveal the whereabouts of the cataract.

There remain a few points of interest which deserve mention. Though in the great majority of couched eyes the cataract lies in the lowest part of the globe, it may be found either to the inner or to the outer side, or even in the upper half of the eye. Sometimes it flaps backward and forward with the movements of the globe, swinging on a hinge, which evidently consists of the remaining fibres of the suspensory ligament, and which may be situate in any possible direction, though most often it lies below. It will be readily understood that if this hinge is situate below, or to the inner or outer sides, the lens will flap away from the pupil downward, or to the hinged side, as the case may be. It is not inconceivable that, in repeatedly doing so, it may inflict some measure of injury on the neighbouring part of the ciliary body and retina, and may thus excite a local inflammation which will tend in time to tie the cataract permanently in the new position towards which it flaps, away from the pupil. In the event of the hinge being in one of the three directions now under discussion, the cataract will tend to fall forward on to the pupil only when the patient stoops forward, so as to bring his face into the horizontal plane. When the hinge is situate above, the latter is one of the few positions of the face in which the pupil clears itself in ordinary cases; but one meets with instances in which, despite the hinge being above, the pupil remains clear except when the face is horizontal, the lens lying most of the time in the upper segment of the eye. There is another factor, and probably a more frequent one, than that of the local injury inflicted by the lens during its movement, which tends to tether it *in situ*. This is the increasing consistence of the vitreous, due to the deposit within it of inflammatory matter, a point which has already been alluded to.

Our next consideration is that of the **cases in which the cataract still lies behind the pupil.** It then seldom, if ever, is in absolutely normal position, and it very frequently is found to have been moved bodily downwards or to one side, or obliquely. Again, but more rarely, it may be tilted backward at an angle with the plane of its normal position. In a great number of cases the history will help one, and, even when the patient denies couching, he will very often admit to having had " medicine applied to his eye by a native practitioner." Should no such evidence be forthcoming, there may still remain that of the lesions to the cornea, the sclera, or the iris, to which attention has already been directed in the previous section.

From these cases we pass on to consider **those in which the lens cannot be seen at all, owing to the occlusion of the pupil.** Here our difficulties are greater still, and, if the history fails us, we must fall back on a careful search for signs of wound scars in the cornea or sclera, or of tears in the iris. A point which is always suggestive is the existence of a cataract in the opposite eye. In such cases as these, the contents of the chamber may be found to consist of pus or of blood.

Our next group is a still more difficult one, for in it **no fundus reflex can be obtained.** It embraces a number of conditions which may be shortly dealt with in turn: (1) Those in which the vitreous body has been converted into a more or less highly organised inflammatory exudate, which is impenetrable to the light of the ophthalmoscope. (2) Those in which this vitreous exudate has contracted inflammatory adhesions to the retina, and by its shrinkage has determined the total detachment of that membrane. (3) Those in which the vitreous chamber has become filled with blood. It is obvious that in all such cases our main dependence must be upon the history, though the other indications already outlined may help us in some of them.

Lastly there are the cases **in which the eye is undergoing shrinkage,** and those in which **phthisis bulbi** is following panophthalmitis. The history of the signs and symptoms of severe iridocyclitis or of suppuration will, in India at least, always excite a suspicion of couching having been performed, unless the patient has a definite story to tell of some other form of injury. Strangely enough, the inventive faculty of the Indian patient does not rise to the height of vamping a narrative of the kind. If he has had an injury, he tells of it readily. If he has been couched, he stolidly denies that anything occurred to cause his trouble, which he states " simply came of itself."

It will be observed that in the preceding remarks we have dealt with two of the problems which confront us in diagnosis, for the simple reason that it is very difficult to separate them; to do so would mean needless repetition. The discovery of the new position of the lens, and of the degree of fixation, if any, it has undergone, can hardly be divorced from the question of whether a couching has or has not been performed. Our third problem was to decide whether it is advisable to operate in any cases, and if so, in which. The Baron de Wenzel, in his treatise on cataract,* records two cases in which his father successfully extracted couched lenses. A number of Anglo-Indian surgeons have had similar experiences, but most of them are reluctant to interfere with these cases oftener than they can help, because, should the operation fail, it is extremely likely that they will unjustly incur the odium for the loss of the patient's vision. On this subject Maynard wrote (*Ophthalmic Review*, April, 1903): " It may be justifiable to attempt the removal of a recently couched lens. If not recent, and more especially if the lens is fixed, it is wiser to leave it alone, even

* Translation by James Ware, surgeon, F.R.S.; London, 1812.

if the sight is failing." To the writer's mind, the one crying indication for removal of a couched lens is that it flaps across and obstructs the pupil. He agrees strongly with Maynard, that if the lens is fixed it is better left alone; but he is doubtful whether the time element is of very great importance, in comparison with the mobility of the cataract ; for a study of the fifty-four globes already dealt with has shown him that the fixation or otherwise of the lens is a question of the amount of septic action set up by the operation. If this is small, the lens may continue mobile, even for a very long period; if it is more severe, the latter will soon be tethered. Dealing with this subject five years ago (Proc. of S. Indian Branch of B.M.A., March 13, 1912), the author wrote as follows:

"We are extremely reluctant in Madras to undertake further operative procedures on an eye in which couching has been performed. Removal of a lens dislocated into the posterior chamber obviously means a wide opening up of the vitreous; and even if the immediate result appears good, there is little guarantee that the benefit will continue. Of eighteen cases in which the lens was removed, twelve obtained better vision at the time, four remained *in statu quo,* and two were rendered worse. I cannot but think that these statistics would suffer if the cases were followed for some years. On five occasions we undertook the laceration of an after-cataract which blocked the line of sight after couching. In two cases there was considerable benefit, whilst in three vision remained *in statu quo antea*. In four cases an iridectomy was performed for optical purposes. In two vision improved slightly, whilst in the two others it remained as before.

"Personally I have a strong and growing objection to undertake any operative procedure on a couched eye. Firstly, there is the risk of lighting up a septic explosion, for which the real responsibility lies with the coucher's original operation; and, secondly, there is the danger of being saddled with the discredit which is justly due to another man's failure."

Reviewing these paragraphs in the light of the much better knowledge of the pathology of couching which we possess to-day, he would urge that only freely movable cataracts should be touched, since want of mobility is associated with profound changes in the vitreous due to septic action. The object that a surgeon sets before him, work where he may, is ever the same —"The greatest good of the greatest number." Failure in such cases as these may play into the hands of the coucher, and enable him to extend his sphere of influence at the expense of the beneficent work of the Western hospitals. The problem in India is a difficult one, in which surgical considerations do not stand alone, but are interwoven with social, moral, and even political questions. Each surgeon must decide for himself what line he will take, and follow it fearlessly.

In this connection, Major Kirkpatrick's experience * in Madras is of considerable value, for he has removed a number of couched lenses, and has been "struck by the rarity of vitreous escape, even after fairly extensive investiga tion with a spoon," during this operation. He adds: "I have noticed that the vitreous body becomes shrunken and extraordinarily tough, so much so that, when an eye is excised (either for glaucoma or for iridocyclitis following Mahomedan operation), the whole globe can be held up by a strabismus hook transfixing the vitreous, though the latter appears perfectly clear. The vitreous undoubtedly does undergo shrinkage, and leaves a large space, which is occupied by aqueous." It is plain that he is referring here to cases in which the vitreous body has undergone some measure of inflammatory organisation, which might be expected to limit the mobility of the lens, and it will be of great interest to learn whether the conclusions of so reliable and experienced an observer ultimately coincide with the author's, that interference should be confined to those cases in which the movements of the cataract within the vitreous body are noted to be free. Once again, let it be emphasised that there are two distinct questions at issue—one the benefit of the individual patient, and the other the good name of Western surgery. Each man must be guided according to the dictates of his own personality and of his environment.

* Personal communication.

CHAPTER VII

CLINICAL

THERE are, in connection with cases of couched cataract, some points of clinical interest which will repay closer attention. These will now be dealt with in turn.

Pain.—The pain which follows the operation of couching has attracted the attention of surgeons from very early times, and there has been much speculation as to its cause. When, after Daviel's discovery, extraction came into serious competition with the older operation, surgeons discussed at much length the relative merit of the two procedures, and it was strongly urged by the extractionists that their operation gave rise to less pain than that of couching. The subject is a very difficult one, for no surgeon, who has had a large cataract practice, can fail to have been struck by the extraordinary difference in the statements of patients as to the amount of suffering they have endured during the first twenty-four hours after the removal of a lens. The majority of them confess to a good deal of pain; this comes on as the effect of the anæsthetic wears off, reaches a maximum, and then slowly dies away, leaving them at the end of twelve hours, and often even at the end of six hours, comparatively comfortable. Occasionally, but rarely, the report is that the pain has been negligible throughout. On the other hand, a bitter complaint of very severe pain is sometimes encountered; fortunately such an occurrence is infrequent. In the case sheets on which the writer's 780 cases were taken, a special heading was provided for notes on the pain inflicted at or after operation. A striking feature of the replies given was the extraordinary difference between them; this is the more astonishing because in a large number of the operations it is probable that no anæsthetic of any kind was used, and yet it was by no means uncommon to meet with patients, who made little or nothing of the pain either at the operation or after it. On the other hand, some complained of terrible suffering, commencing as soon as the needle was inserted, and lasting for long periods thereafter. The majority admitted to some pain, but neither belittled nor exaggerated it. It will thus be seen that, so far as pain is concerned, the experiences of the coucher and of the extractor are much alike; it is unfair to judge either operation on exceptional cases.

Looking at the subject from the anatomical side, the writer is bound to confess that an argument *a priori* would have led him to expect extraction to have been by far the more painful of the two procedures, both at the time and during the early hours of convalescence, although much has been made by early writers of injury to the retina and to the sensitive ciliary body, and of the extensive damage done by the needle during a couching. We know, however, that injury to the retina does not produce pain; and we are also well aware of the extreme susceptibility of the cornea to pain. Surely the extent of damage inflicted on sensitive structures is, as a rule, much greater in an extraction than it is in a couching. How then are we to explain the dread with which surgeons, in the days of couching, looked forward to the suffering and vomiting which sometimes followed the operation? In answer to this question the following suggestions are put forward. The pain of the first twelve hours is to be sharply differentiated from that which begins on the second or third day, always remembering, however, that, though the causes are different, the one may run into the other. The early pain may be ascribed (1) to injury to the nerves of the ciliary body and iris, especially when the laceration of those structures is considerable, as our clinical experience and our specimens alike show it sometimes is; (2) to hæmorrhage from the vessels of the ciliary body, the iris, the choroid or the retina: such hæmorrhage may produce pain in two ways—(*a*) by dissecting up sensitive structures, and (*b*) by increasing the tension of the eye; and (3) to the rapid production of early glaucoma. There are several ways in which we may conceive that such a glaucoma might be produced. We have already mentioned the possibility of hæmorrhage. Then we have to remember that, in the course of this operation, the anterior portion of the vitreous body is often extensively interfered with. It is conceivable that a forward movement of this part may close the angle of the chamber, and so interfere with excretion. Again, when the lens is forced back on the vitreous body, and the anterior hyaloid layer remains unbroken, we sometimes find it acting as a wedge, pushing the base of the iris forward, and thrusting the hyaloid membrane backward. The latter action must press on the vitreous body, and so make it bulge at other parts of the circumference of the eye, thus tending to close the angle of filtration over such areas. It is obvious that the pressure of the lens on the iris base will directly close the sinus locally to a greater or less degree. A point that we must never lose sight of is that the very great majority of these patients are in the glaucoma period of life, and with a certain number of them very little alteration of the *status quo* is required to precipitate an attack of pathological high tension. If we take all these factors into account, and especially if we bear in mind the great variability that different patients present in their sensibility to pain, we shall have little difficulty in understanding that couching may sometimes be followed within the first few hours by great suffering attended with vomiting.

When we come to discuss the later pain, all difficulty vanishes. The frequency with which iridocyclitis and glaucoma dog the footsteps of couching in India, explains at once the bitter and oft-repeated history of pain coming on within the first two or three days, and lasting for months or even for years.

Some Rare Accidents following Couching.—In a large series of cases such as we now have under review, it was to be expected that some unusual incidents would be met with. A few of these will be dealt with.

1. *The Dislocation of the Lens into the Anterior Chamber.*—This accident was known to the early writers. It may occur either at the time of operation or subsequently. In the former case the nucleus alone may be dislocated, or the whole lens may be driven forward in its capsule. It may lie loose and freely movable in the chamber, or may become mechanically impacted there, or, lastly, may be firmly fixed *in situ* as a result of inflammatory action. In the cases of late dislocation it is usually

the nucleus alone that passes forward, the cortex having either become absorbed or the cataract having originally been of the Morgagnian variety. Such are the cases which give rise to the interesting clinical phenomenon of a nucleus which passes backwards and forwards between the two chambers. In some cases alterations in the position of the patient's head suffice to make the lens travel in one direction or the other.

2. *The Dislocation of the Lens between the Ciliary Body and the Sclera* through the ruptured pectinate ligament occurred in one case. Such an accident must be very rare under any possible conditions of eye injury. J. B. Lawford, in the Reports of the Royal London Ophthalmic Hospital (1886-87, p. 334), recorded a similar happening which followed a blow on the eye by a clasp-knife thrown at a woman. Nettleship (Ophth. Soc. Trans., vol. i.) also published a case in which an opaque lens disappeared into a pouch between the choroid and sclera when the patient lay down, and reappeared in the anterior chamber when he stood up. The condition followed a blow on the eye inflicted some years previously.

3. *Dislocation of the Lens behind the Retina.*—This accident was known to the early writers, and Mackenzie expressly gives the warning that, if in effecting depression " the handle of the needle is raised much higher than the horizontal position, the cataract is apt to be pressed through the retina, and vision extinguished." Daviel had met with the same condition in eyes which he dissected after death, and which had been couched by other surgeons. We, too, encountered it twice in our pathological material. In one eye the retina had been torn away from the ora serrata, and the lens pushed behind it; in the other, an extensive hole had been torn in the retina, and through this the cataract had been thrust. In both, the cataracts were Morgagnian and had been dislocated in their capsules, and in both, the retinæ had undergone total detachment, in this latter respect testifying to the value of Mackenzie's warning.

A Comparison of Depression and Reclination.—There can be no question that the operation of reclination breaks up the vitreous body to a considerably greater extent than mere depression of the cataract does. On the other hand, the claim is made that after its performance the lens is much less likely to undergo reascension; indeed, it was for this reason that Willburg introduced the method; and, if we may judge from the evidence of later writers, he was justified by results. So far as the Indian coucher is concerned, it seems a little doubtful whether he has any clear conception of the difference between the two procedures; indeed, so long as he gets the lens out of the way of the pupil, it is probable that he neither knows nor cares which method he has succeeded in adopting, though he probably much more often reclines than depresses. This may be explained by the experience of a number of European surgeons, that it is more easy to effect reclination than depression. An interesting point is that in quite a number of our pathological specimens the lens lay in front of the anterior hyaloid membrane, and therefore outside the vitreous body; most of these were cases of depression, but in a few of them the lens is turned backwards at an angle with its ordinary plane, clearly showing that a partial reclination had been effected.

Reascension of Couched Cataract.—This subject has been partly dealt with in the preceding paragraphs. Naturally, it was a topic which attracted a good deal of attention from the early writers, who commented on its relative frequency immediately after the operation, and gave elaborate instructions to prevent its occurrence. Some of them went so far as to suggest the frequent repetition of the operation, if necessary. In their experience it would appear that, if reascension failed to occur within the first fortnight, the prospect of the lens remaining down was good. Nevertheless, they were familiar with the fact that, even after years of a happy result, the cataract might suddenly be found to have returned to its old position opposite the pupil. In some cases this misfortune followed a blow or fall on the head, or a severe jar of the whole body. Similar stories may be heard in an Indian out-patient room to-day. This is a point which must be taken well into consideration by any who think fit to resort to couching in selected cases.

A Comparison of the Corneal and Scleral Routes for Operation.—It has been already shown that the Indian operators of the present day vary in their technique, some attacking the lens from in front through the cornea, and others from behind through the sclera. It is interesting to note that there is a similar difference in practice amongst those of the modern surgeons who have adopted couching in special cases. There can, however, be no doubt that the weight of opinion among the old writers was all in favour of the posterior operation; and Mackenzie, whose practical experience was, we may hope, vastly greater than that of any modern surgeon, summed up the position in these words: " In this way (*i.e.*, through the cornea) neither operation (depression or reclination) can be satisfactorily performed." We may close this subject with another word of warning to any who are inclined to favour the couching of lenses in selected cases. From the time of Celsus onwards, surgeons who have had large experience in couching have warned their disciples that it is an operation much more easy to undertake than to carry to a successful technical issue, and have cautioned them against venturing on it until they have seen it performed many times at the hands of an expert. One cannot conclude better than by a quotation from the writings of Lieut.-Colonel Henry Smith, who has had very large opportunities of observing the results of cataract couching. He is known to be a very skilful operator, and one, therefore, who is little likely to exaggerate the difficulties of any ophthalmic procedure, yet he writes: " It is no easy matter to completely dislocate the lens, and, in my observation, the partial dislocation is more frequent than the complete in the hands of adepts of the art."

The Dislocation of Morgagnian Cataracts.—A curious error is to be found pervading many of the early writings on couching—viz., that a Morgagnian cataract could not be couched in its capsule. Our hospital experience in India proved that this idea was erroneous, and the examination of our pathological specimens has shown the correctness of our clinical deductions. The Morgagnian lens may be dislocated forward into the anterior chamber, backward into the vitreous, and even through the coats of the retina, without rupture of its capsule. This is far from being a surprise to any surgeon who has operated on a number of these cases, for the Morgagnian capsule is usually very much tougher than that of any other form of cataract. It has already been mentioned that, if the capsule bursts, the nucleus may escape, and may then sometimes be found either floating freely in one of the chambers of the eye, or fixed in one position by inflammatory adhesions, or, still more rarely, passing from chamber to chamber at intervals. The writer has observed that in some cases the escape of Morgagnian fluid into an eye appears to cause great irritation. The same fact has been observed by some of the early writers on couching.

INDEX